WITHDRAWN
WRIGHT STATE UNIVERSITY LIBRARIES

An Introduction to the Life and Work of John Hughlings Jackson with a Catalogue Raisonné of his Writings

(*Medical History*, Supplement No. 26)

An Introduction to the Life and Work of John Hughlings Jackson with a Catalogue Raisonné of his Writings

by

GEORGE K YORK

and

DAVID A STEINBERG

Fiddletown Institute and Kaiser Permanente Stockton
Medical Center, California

(*Medical History*, Supplement No. 26)

London
The Wellcome Trust Centre for the History of Medicine at UCL
2006

© George K York and David A Steinberg 2006

All Rights Reserved. No part of this publication may be reproduced, stored in a retrieval system, or transmitted, in any form or by any means, electronic, mechanical photocopying, recording or otherwise, without prior permission.

ISBN 0-85484-109-1; 978-0-85484-109-7

Supplements to *Medical History* may be obtained by post from BMJ Publishing Group, BMA House, Tavistock Square, London WC1H 9JR, UK; and the Wellcome Library, 210 Euston Road, London NW1 2BE, UK.

Contents

Preface	vii
An Introduction to the Life and Work of John Hughlings Jackson	1
Biographical Sketch	3
Hughlings Jackson's Neurological Method	9
The Nature of the Epileptic Discharge	12
Jacksonian Epilepsy	13
Cerebral Localization	15
The Sensorimotor Machine	16
Weighted Ordinal Representation	17
Evolutionary Neurophysiology	19
The Doctrine of Concomitance	20
The Rejection of the Unconscious	21
Aphasia	24
Recovery	25
Ophthalmology in its Relation to General Medicine	27
Hughlings Jackson's Philosophy	28
The Bibliography of John Hughlings Jackson	30
Catalogue Raisonné of the Writings of John Hughlings Jackson	35
Appendix 1: Pamphlets of John Hughlings Jackson, Rockefeller Medical Library, Institute of Neurology, UCL	140
Appendix 2: Unpublished Manuscripts of John Hughlings Jackson, Rockefeller Medical Library, Institute of Neurology, UCL	146
Index	151

Preface

As junior doctors, one of us watched as consultant neurologists evaluated patients with neurological diseases while the other investigated the mathematics and physics of the new imaging technologies. Computerized imaging was in the process of development, and professors of neurology were the product of classical training that depended on clinical diagnosis. They took great pains to elicit a detailed history, then engaged in a ritualized set of bedside manoeuvres that, to an uninitiated observer, would seem almost magical, and certainly inexplicable. Nevertheless, they arrived at a correct diagnosis with remarkable frequency.

At the same time we were reading the history of physics, chemistry and mathematics. These histories, which often took the form of scientific biographies, made us curious about the origins of the strange science of diagnostic neurology. When we examined neurology in the nineteenth and twentieth century, we found that many people made crucial observations about the anatomy, physiology and pathology of the nervous system. On the other hand, we were surprised to find that the conceptual threads of our research consistently led us to the work of John Hughlings Jackson. This confluence motivated us to embark on a detailed study of Hughlings Jackson's ideas.

Like most students, we began with the papers collected in the *Selected writings of John Hughlings Jackson*, edited by his amanuensis James Taylor. When we started to think seriously about the circumstances under which Hughlings Jackson worked, we recognized that the *Selected writings* are completely devoid of context or commentary. We also realized that, though the *Selected writings* are printed to a high standard of accuracy, Taylor edited and combined papers in ways that obscure an understanding of the development of Hughlings Jackson's ideas. We therefore undertook to collect and categorize Hughlings Jackson's writings by examining them in their primary states: as articles printed in the medical literature of 1861–1911. This resulted in the catalogue raisonné that we present here. We have been able to find eighty-four previously unrecognized works by and about Hughlings Jackson.

Our introduction to the life and works of Hughlings Jackson is intended to guide readers through the development of his neurological ideas, and to provide the most accurate bibliography of his work. We have only hinted at its social, medical, scientific and intellectual context, and we acknowledge that this context is a rich source for historical research. We hope that our work will direct Jackson scholars, and general readers, to the original sources for his work.

This study would not have been possible without the invaluable support of librarians and archivists in London and California. We particularly thank Louise Shepherd and Kate Bricknell, at the Rockefeller Library of the Institute of Neurology, University College London, and Jonathan Evans at the Royal London Hospital. We thank the librarians at the University of California in Davis and San Francisco, Stanford University, the California State Library, and the Royal Society of Medicine in London. We also thank our wives, Pamela Wehrlie York and Tracy K Genesen, for their patience and support.

George K York
David A Steinberg

Fiddletown CA
23 December 2005

An Introduction to the Life and Work of John Hughlings Jackson

Introduction

In 1860, physicians had no systematic procedure for diagnosing diseases of the nervous system. Even worse, they had no conceptual basis by which to organize their thinking about how the nervous system works. By 1910, they were able to diagnose neurological disease using consistent scientific principles. The development of scientific neurology is a model of how science emerges.

John Hughlings Jackson created the conceptual framework for clinical neurophysiology, the discipline that underlies diagnostic neurology. He began by establishing a consistent scientific method based on the systematic analysis of anatomy, pathology and physiology. This method revolved around his concept of the focal lesion, a concept that he refined and which became a cornerstone of bedside neurology. He recognized that focal epilepsy and focal necrosis can be viewed as reciprocal physiological processes, and concluded that somatotopic representation is found in the entire nervous system including the cortex.

Hughlings Jackson was a practising physician with little formal education in non-medical topics. His practical framework for thinking about neurophysiology applied contemporaneous evolutionary theories to medicine. He conceived of diseases of the nervous system as a process of de-evolution, or dissolution. He came to believe that the nervous system is hierarchy of three evolutionary levels that represent, re-represent and re-re-represent movement and sensation of the parts of the body. Higher levels suppress the function of lower levels, so that the symptoms of neurological disease are dual in nature. Negative symptoms result from the loss of function of higher levels, and positive symptoms result from the appearance of the function of previously inhibited lower levels. These emergent functions are inherently less organized, less definite and more general than the functions that are lost.

Physicians admired Hughlings Jackson during his lifetime, but his personality and the nature of his work made him invisible to the larger scientific and cultural world. The appearance of experimental and cognitive neuroscience in the twentieth century has made his ideas more widely influential, and there is every reason to think that this trend will continue.

Biographical Sketch

John Hughlings Jackson was born on 4 April 1835 at Providence Green, his father's home in Green Hammerton, ten miles northwest of the city of York. He was the youngest of five children, with three brothers and a sister. His father, Samuel Jackson, was a prosperous brewer and farmer. His mother, the former Sarah Hughlings, was the daughter of John Hughlings, an excise collector from Northowram in west Yorkshire. John Hughlings Jackson was baptised on 19 June 1835 in the Independent Chapel of Green Hammerton

Introduction

by his great-uncle, the dissenting minister James Jackson. His mother died when he was a year old.[1]

He was educated at the local school in Green Hammerton, followed by stints at boarding schools in Tadcaster, in Yorkshire, and Nailsworth, in Gloucestershire.[2] He attended school with his older brother Thomas, who supported and encouraged him during his childhood and for whom he retained a lifelong affection. On 20 October 1850, aged fifteen, he ended his formal education and became an apprentice to Dr William Charles Anderson and his son Tempest Anderson, prosperous physicians who lived at 23 Stonegate in York.[3]

After two years of working in the Anderson household, Hughlings Jackson began classes at the York Medical School, where William Anderson was a lecturer.[4] The faculty, made up of local practitioners, lectured for a fee to the dozen or so students in attendance. Here he was a student of Thomas Laycock, later professor of medicine at Edinburgh, who exerted a strong influence on his career and on his medical and physiological interests.[5]

In order to practise general medicine in Yorkshire, he had to qualify as a surgeon and apothecary. The Apothecaries Act of 1815 required candidates for their licence to present evidence of attendance at an approved hospital, and the York County Hospital was just such an institution. The Worshipful Society of Apothecaries accepted Hughlings Jackson's training in York as a qualification for their licence, and on 10 April 1856, he presented himself at the Apothecaries Hall for examination.[6] The record of this purely oral examination gives his place of residence as Green Hammerton, Yorkshire. He presented his apprenticeship indenture and a testimonial of his moral character from William Anderson, and evidence of his attendance at the required course of lectures at the York Medical School. Completing this examination successfully, he took the qualification LSA.[7]

In order to qualify for membership, the Royal College of Surgeons required a year's attendance on a surgical ward of a large hospital in addition to attendance at lectures. No hospital in York was acceptable to the Royal College; hence in 1855 and 1856 Hughlings Jackson walked the wards at St Bartholomew's Hospital in London. Even though he was one among many medical students, his performance attracted the attention of James Paget.[8]

---

[1] For biographical details, consult James Taylor's biographical memoir in John Hughlings Jackson, *Neurological Fragments*, London, Oxford University Press, 1925, pp. 1–26. See also Macdonald Critchley and Eileen A Critchley, *John Hughlings Jackson: father of English Neurology*, Oxford, Oxford University Press, 1998.

[2] Taylor, op. cit., note 1 above, p. 2.

[3] MS 8241/18, fol. 58, no. 7 in the Society of Apothecaries' Court of Examiners' Candidates' Entry Book (1855–1858), which is a microfilm of a document located in the Guildhall library, London. See also the seminal study by Samuel H Greenblatt, 'The major influences on the early life and work of John Hughlings Jackson', *Bull Hist Med*, 1965, **39**: 346–376, pp. 347 note 3.

[4] J H Wetherill, 'The York Medical School', *Med Hist*, 1961, **5**: 253–269, p. 257.

[5] For an overview of Laycock's life and work, see Michael Barfoot, *"To ask the suffrages of the patrons": Thomas Laycock and the Edinburgh chair of medicine, 1855*, London, Wellcome Institute for the History of Medicine, 1995, pp. 1–22.

[6] Society of Apothecaries' Court of Examiners' Candidates' Entry Book (1855–1858), op. cit., note 3 above, p. 58, no. 7. This licence would not have allowed Hughlings Jackson to practise in the City of London or within a seven-mile radius of it. See also S W F Holloway, 'The Apothecaries' Act, 1815: a reinterpretation. Part I: The origins of the Act', *Med Hist*, 1966, **10**: 107–29, pp. 124–125, and 'The Apothecaries' Act, 1815: a reinterpretation. Part II: The consequences of the Act', *Med Hist*, 1966, **10**: 221–236, p. 233.

[7] See MS 8241/18, fol. 58, in the Society of Apothecaries' Court of Examiners' Candidates' Entry Book (1855–1858), op. cit., note 3 above.

[8] 'London Hospital. Presentation of testimonial to Dr. Hughlings Jackson, F.R.S., by Sir James Paget', *Br Med J*, 1895, **ii**: 861–863.

Introduction

In 1856 Hughlings Jackson passed the examination of the Royal College of Surgeons, although no records remain of his performance in the examination, and took the qualification MRCS.

The qualifications of the Surgeons' College and the Apothecaries' Hall entitled him to practise as a surgeon-apothecary and, as LSA and MRCS, he could have returned to Yorkshire to seek his fortune as a general practitioner.[9] His alternative was to seek further training and to qualify as a physician. He might have sought a Continental or Scottish education with the aim of taking an MD, but he took another road, one that was at once more familiar and safer. He stayed in Yorkshire.

Hughlings Jackson had other reasons for returning to Yorkshire. His father had suffered serious financial reverses, possibly by speculating in railway stock. The precise timing of Samuel Jackson's financial troubles is not clear, but in a letter dated 17 March 1854 Samuel Jackson exhorted his son John to a life of frugality in dress and custom.[10] Hughlings Jackson's three brothers emigrated to New Zealand after 1856, at the same time that their father moved out of Providence Green and into a house in Green Hammerton. His father was by now not only impoverished but in failing health, which may have motivated Hughlings Jackson's return in 1856. On 9 February 1858 Samuel Jackson died; his son John was in his second year as a houseman in York.

After qualifying, he was appointed resident medical officer at the York Dispensary and spent the next three years as a house officer. Little is known of this phase of his medical training, but we do know that he endured personal reverses, beginning with the emigration of his brothers. His sister Ann, never in good health, had a stroke, and died in 1859. Thus, by the end of his house years he was left with no close family in the country.[11]

While he was a houseman he joined the York Medical Society, whose minute book contains his first recorded analysis of diseases of the nervous system. In this report, dated 8 January 1859, Hughlings Jackson presented cases of paralysis arising from diseases of the spine, corpus striatum and hemispheres.[12] In his discussion, Hughlings Jackson referred to the ideas of Robert Bentley Todd, indicating that he was familiar with Todd's volume of lectures on paralysis and other diseases of the nervous system.

At some time between May and October 1859 Hughlings Jackson left the city of York and moved to London.[13] He carried an introduction to his fellow Yorkshireman Jonathan Hutchinson, with whom he soon formed a lifelong friendship. Nearly seven years older than Hughlings Jackson, Hutchinson had followed a similar path into London medicine. In the summer of 1859 Hutchinson was a member of the medical staff at a number of London hospitals, including the Royal London Ophthalmic Hospital and the London Hospital.[14]

---

[9] M Jeanne Peterson, *The medical profession in mid-Victorian London*, Berkeley, University of California Press, 1978, p. 11.

[10] Critchley and Critchley, op. cit., note 1 above, pp. 29–31.

[11] Ibid., pp. 1–32.

[12] Greenblatt cites this document as being in the Minute Book 1844–1870. MS in the library of the York Medical Society. See Greenblatt, op. cit., note 3 above, pp. 350–351.

[13] Ibid., p. 351.

[14] See Herbert Hutchinson's quotations from his father's diary entries in Herbert Hutchinson, *Jonathan Hutchinson: life and letters*, London, William Heinemann Medical Books, 1946, pp. 21–26. See also 'Obituary. Sir Jonathan Hutchinson, F.R.C.S., F.R.S.', *Br Med J*, 1913, **i**: 1398–1401, p. 1398.

Introduction

From 1859, Hughlings Jackson lived with Hutchinson and his family at 4 Finsbury Circus, London. Through Hutchinson's influence, the younger man was appointed Physician to the Metropolitan Free Hospital and the Royal London Ophthalmic Hospital in 1859. In the same year he began his long association with the London Hospital with an appointment as lecturer in pathology.

In September 1860 Hughlings Jackson travelled to Scotland and presented himself for examination for the MD of the University of St Andrews. Licentiates of the Society of Apothecaries and Members of the Royal College of Surgeons were eligible to become candidates for the degree. On payment of the graduation fee of twenty-five guineas, the candidate could sit three days of written examination followed by an oral examination. The candidates were required to provide a written translation from the first four books of Celsus, to write prescriptions in Latin and to be able to interpret medical and scientific terms derived from Greek. In addition, they answered written questions on clinical topics.[15] On 28 September 1860 a panel of the faculty examined Hughlings Jackson personally. Having satisfied the panel, the degree MD St Andrews was conferred on him on 28 September 1860.[16]

Hutchinson and Hughlings Jackson were bright and ambitious young doctors, anxious to make their mark on the metropolis. First Hutchinson, then Hughlings Jackson, became medical reporters for the weekly *Medical Times and Gazette*. In the 14 July 1860 number, Jonathan Hutchinson began a by-lined column entitled 'Reports of hospital practice in medicine and surgery'.[17] From 19 January 1861 this column carried the joint by-line of Jonathan Hutchinson and John Hughlings Jackson.[18] It was rare to have a by-lined column in a weekly medical journal in that era, so the two Yorkshiremen could achieve a degree of notoriety in London medicine. As reporters, they attended lectures and rounds in the teaching hospitals of London, where their presence would have been noticed, even cultivated, by physicians anxious for a favourable public comment.

One such physician was Charles Edouard Brown-Séquard, the pioneering neurophysiologist and founding physician at the National Hospital for the Paralysed and Epileptic, Queen Square. An important influence on Hughlings Jackson, Brown-Séquard taught the primacy of physiology in medical science, an attitude that became central to Hughlings Jackson's scientific thinking. He also advised Hughlings Jackson to specialize in diseases of the nervous system.[19] In 1861 Hughlings Jackson passed the examination for Membership of the Royal College of Physicians, and on 7 May 1862 he was appointed Assistant Physician at the Hospital for the Paralysed and Epileptic, proposed by Brown-Séquard. On

---

[15] See Irvine Loudon, *Medical care and the general practitioner, 1750–1850*, Oxford, Clarendon, 1986, pp. 214–227, and also J A Shepherd, 'Medical teaching at St. Andrews University 1413–1972', *Br Med J*, 1972, **iii**: 38–41.

[16] Records of the University of St Andrews. The Critchleys write that Hughlings Jackson submitted a thesis in support of his degree, but we could find no trace of such a thesis, which was in any case not required for the degree. See Critchley and Critchley, op. cit., note 1 above, p. 33.

[17] Jonathan Hutchinson, 'Reports of hospital practice in medicine and surgery', *Med Times Gaz*, 1860, **ii**: 31–34.

[18] Jonathan Hutchinson and John Hughlings Jackson, 'Reports of hospital practice in medicine and surgery', *Med Times Gaz*, 1861, **i**: 60–63.

[19] See Jonathan Hutchinson, 'The late Dr. Hughlings Jackson: recollections of a lifelong friendship', *Br Med J*, 1911, **ii**: 1551–1554. For the life and work of Brown-Séquard, consult Michael J Aminoff, *Brown-Séquard: a visionary of science*, New York, Raven Press, 1993.

Introduction

25 August 1863 Hughlings Jackson was appointed Assistant Physician to the London Hospital and in 1874 he became Physician to that hospital.[20]

In June 1864, Hughlings Jackson delivered a lecture at the London Hospital, later published in the London Hospital *Reports*, on the method of diagnostic neurology. This lecture established a system of clinical physiology that endures to this day. That summer he published a series of case analyses in the same journal that provided strong support for Paul Broca's identification of a centre for language in the left inferior frontal lobe.[21] These articles established his reputation as a clinical neurologist.

On 25 July 1865, John Hughlings Jackson married the love of his life, his first cousin Elizabeth Dade Jackson, at St Giles Church, Northampton. Jonathan Hutchinson acted as best man, and described the festivities in a letter to his wife.[22] By all accounts the marriage was a happy one, though Hughlings Jackson complained in a letter to his brother that he was not making as much money as he wanted.[23] In 1866 Hughlings Jackson attended the victims of a cholera epidemic in the East End of London, for which he was awarded a gold watch from the governors of the London Hospital. He was proud of the watch, which he wore for the rest of his life and which now resides in the museum of the London Hospital.[24]

In 1868, aged thirty-three, Hughlings Jackson was elected a Fellow of the Royal College of Physicians, a substantial achievement for someone with no university education. The next year he gave the Goulstonian lectures at the RCP, an honour usually accorded the most distinguished new Fellow. Abstracts of the lectures appeared in both the *Lancet* and the *British Medical Journal* in February and March 1869.[25] In these lectures he applied the method he had announced at the London Hospital in 1864 to the study of hemiplegia. He pointed out that hemiplegia and lateralized seizures were physiologically reciprocal states. He also said that the general scientific world would look to medicine for an explanation of the function of the nervous system and the relationship of the brain and the mind.[26]

The London establishment sometimes lampooned the University of St Andrews because it awarded degrees to those who could pay the fee and pass the examination. To burnish its claim to scientific credibility, the St Andrews Medical Graduates Association published

---

[20] See 'Obituary. John Hughlings Jackson, M.D., F.R.C.P., F.R.S.', *Br Med J*, 1911, **ii**: 950–954, p. 950, and 'Obituary. John Hughlings Jackson, M.D. St. And., F.R.C.P. Lond., LL.D., D.Sc.,F.R.S.', *Lancet*, 1911, **ii**: 1103–1107.

[21] See J Hughlings Jackson, 'On the study of diseases of the nervous system. A lecture delivered June, 1864', *Clinical Lectures and Reports by the Medical and Surgical Staff of the London Hospital*, 1864, **1**: 146–158, and also J Hughlings Jackson, 'Loss of speech: its association with valvular disease of the heart, and with hemiplegia on the right side.—Defects of smell.—Defects of speech in chorea.—Arterial regions in epilepsy', *Clinical Lectures and Reports by the Medical and Surgical Staff of the London Hospital*, 1864, **1**: 388–471.

[22] See Herbert Hutchinson, op. cit., note 14 above, p. 229.

[23] Letter quoted in Critchley and Critchley, op. cit., note 1 above, p. 173.

[24] See Taylor, op. cit., note 1 above, p. 22, and also Critchley and Critchley, op. cit., note 1 above, pp. 41–43.

[25] See J Hughlings Jackson, 'Abstract of the Gulstonian [sic] lectures on certain points in the study and classification of diseases of the nervous system. Delivered at the Royal College of Physicians', *Lancet*, 1869, **i**: 307–308, 344–345, 379–380, and 'Gulstonian lectures on certain points in the study and classification of diseases of the nervous system. Delivered at the Royal College of Physicians', *Br Med J*, 1869, **i**: 184, 210, and 236.

[26] See *Lancet*, ibid., p. 307.

Introduction

yearly transactions between 1867 and 1873. In the 1869 *Transactions*, printed in 1870, Hughlings Jackson published his pivotal 'A study of convulsions', in which he described the physiology of focal epilepsy, and the localization that can result.[27]

The 1870s were a time of accomplishment, acclaim and personal sorrow for Hughlings Jackson. Based on clinical observations of the march of myoclonic jerks in partial epilepsy, he concluded that parts of the body were represented in discrete parts of the nervous system. His system of somatotopic organization applied to both sensory and motor systems, and was dramatically confirmed by Gustav Fritsch and Eduard Hitzig's demonstration of the electrical excitability of the motor cortex of dogs.[28] Hitzig acknowledged Hughlings Jackson's achievement, which led to Hughlings Jackson's international scientific acclaim. At the same time his investigation of the workings of the nervous system led him to contemporaneous evolutionary theory. Between October 1874 and December 1876, he published a series of articles on the diagnosis of epilepsy in which he set out the principles of his theory of evolutionary neurophysiology.[29]

Amid this intense intellectual activity Hughlings Jackson experienced his deepest personal sorrow when, on 25 May 1876, Elizabeth Dade Jackson died unexpectedly. James Taylor, Hughlings Jackson's student, collaborator, biographer and unofficial secretary, tells us that Mrs. Jackson died of cerebral venous thrombosis complicated by Jacksonian focal seizures.[30] Hughlings Jackson was shattered at the loss of his beloved companion, and remained emotionally stricken for the rest of his life.

In 1878, aged forty-three, he received an important scientific honour when he was elected a Fellow of the Royal Society. Also in 1878 he joined John Charles Bucknill, James Crichton-Browne and David Ferrier as founding editors of the journal *Brain*. In March 1884 he delivered the Croonian lectures at the Royal College of Physicians on the topic of evolution and dissolution of the nervous system, a seminal moment in scientific neurology.[31] In these lectures he articulated his mature conception of disease of the nervous system as a process of de-evolution, or dissolution. In this conception, the nervous system is a hierarchy of sensorimotor centres whose connections are governed by evolutionary principles.

For the next fifteen years he wrote, saw patients and participated in medical life in London. Though he is said to have lived a lonely existence after the death of his wife, he was engaged enough in medical affairs to be elected president of the Harveian Society (1886), the Medical Society of London (1887) and the Ophthalmological Society of the United Kingdom (1889). In 1890 he gave the Lumleian lectures on epilepsy at the Royal

---

[27] J Hughlings Jackson, 'A study of convulsions', *St Andrews Medical Graduates' Association Transactions 1869*, 1870, pp. 162–204. See also Owsei Temkin, *The falling sickness*, 2nd ed. rev., Baltimore, Johns Hopkins University Press, 1971, pp. 328–344.

[28] G Fritsch, E Hitzig, 'Über die elektrische Erregbarkeit des Grosshirn', *Archiv für Anatomie, Physiologie und wissenschaftliche Medicin*, 1870: 300–332.

[29] See J Hughlings Jackson, 'On the scientific and empirical investigations of epilepsies', *Med Press Circular*, 1874, **18**: 325–327, 347–352, 389–392, 409–412, 475–478, 497–499, 519–521; 1875, **19**: 353–355, 397–400, 419–421; 1875, **20**: 313–315, 355–358, 487–489; 1876, **21**: 63–65, 129–131, 173–176, 313–316; 1876, **22**: 145–147, 185–187, 475–477.

[30] Taylor, op. cit., note 1 above, p. 15.

[31] J Hughlings Jackson, 'The Croonian lectures on evolution and dissolution of the nervous system. Delivered at the Royal College of Physicians, March, 1884', *Br Med J*, 1884, **i**: 591–593, 660–663, 703–707.

Introduction

College of Physicians, becoming one of the few physicians ever honoured by the Goulstonian, Croonian and Lumleian lectureships. He was a member of the Council of the Royal College of Physicians from 1885 to 1887, and a Censor of the College from 1888 to 1889.[32] In 1885 he was elected the first President of the Neurological Society of London, by acclamation, and gave the first Hughlings Jackson Lecture of that society on 8 December 1897.[33] He received honorary degrees from the universities of Edinburgh and Glasgow and Bologna. He was particularly pleased by his honorary degree from the University of Bologna, in respect of the ancient medical traditions of that university. He was awarded an honorary Doctorate of Science upon the opening of the University of Leeds, in his native Yorkshire, an honour of which he was particularly proud.[34]

When Hughlings Jackson retired from the London Hospital in 1894, his testimonial was chaired by the now-knighted Sir James Paget, who praised his former student as an important scientist who regarded the bedside and the laboratory as equally suited for scientific study.[35] His retirement from the National Hospital at the age of sixty-five, in 1900, was postponed five years because of his continuing contributions to neurology. Becoming progressively deaf and reclusive in his old age, he spent most of his time in his house at 3 Manchester Square. He died there, of pneumonia, on 7 October 1911, aged seventy-six years six months.

Hughlings Jackson's Neurological Method

Neurology did not exist as an organized scientific discipline in 1860. Both Todd and Brown-Séquard had medical practices in the 1850s that were mainly composed of patients with neurological diseases, but neurology as a specialty had no institutional structure. The National Hospital, Queen Square, had just been founded, but its medical staff were expected to have simultaneous appointments in general hospitals in the metropolis. Much of the medical establishment held strong biases against specialists and specialty hospitals. At the same time, grand scientific syntheses had gained currency in Victorian England. In this milieu Hughlings Jackson enunciated a practical diagnostic method that formed the basis of bedside neurology for the next hundred years.

As a medical reporter, Hughlings Jackson attended Brown-Séquard's clinical lectures, and he knew Todd's published neurological work. Both Todd and Brown-Séquard analysed cases pre-mortem and at autopsy, and both assumed that the nervous system is an aggregate of anatomically contiguous but physiologically discrete components, or organs. The phrenological assumption originated in the work of Franz Josef Gall, who sought to assess a person's character by palpation of the skull.[36] The explicit analysis of pre-mortem

---

[32] 'Obituary', *Br Med J*, note 20 above, pp. 951–2.
[33] J Hughlings Jackson, 'The Hughlings Jackson lecture on the relations of different divisions of the central nervous system to one another and to parts of the body. Delivered before the Neurological Society, Dec. 8th, 1897', *Lancet*, 1898, **i**: 79–87.
[34] Taylor, op. cit., note 1 above, pp. 21–22.
[35] 'Opening of the winter session in the medical schools. London Hospital. Presentation of testimonial to Dr. Hughlings Jackson, F.R.S., by Sir James Paget', *Br Med J*, 1895, **ii**: 861–863.
[36] Owsei Temkin, 'Gall and the phrenological movement', *Bull Hist Med*, 1947, **21**: 275–321.

Introduction

neurological signs and symptoms, followed by post-mortem inspection of the nervous system, revealed the pathological nature of a number of individual neurological diseases. By determining which neurological organs are affected and which are spared, the physician could predict the location and nature of post-mortem tissue damage. Though the phrenological technique of ascertaining character by palpation of the skull had been discredited, the phrenological assumption that the nervous system is an aggregate of separate organs, each with a distinct function, was embedded in the method of clinico-pathological correlation which characterized neurology in 1860. However, there was as yet no consensus on the definition of neurological function or on the methods to be employed to test those functions at the bedside or in the laboratory.

Hughlings Jackson was dissatisfied with conventional case analysis of patients with neurological disease. In late 1863 he produced his first attempt at a systematic neurophysiology, a privately circulated pamphlet entitled *Suggestions for studying diseases of the nervous system on Professor Owen's vertebral theory*. In the introduction he wrote, "In studying the Natural History of Diseases of the Nervous System, I have experienced great difficulty, not only in arranging notes of cases, but also in thinking of the disease as a lesion of a certain physiological system."[37] He went on to propose a neurophysiological system, based on Richard Owen's vertebral theory, in which each vertebral segment controls a distinct distribution of visceral organs, circulation, dermatome and myotome, all under the control of the cortex. In the preface to this pamphlet, dated 5 January 1863, he said that his interest was not in the details of the system but in understanding how the nervous system worked in health and disease. He wrote, "To sum up, I care very little about the fate of the details of the scheme, and will willingly sacrifice all of them, if I can make a better arrangement."[38]

In June 1864 Hughlings Jackson mounted the podium at the London Hospital to deliver a lecture entitled 'On the study of diseases of the nervous system'.[39] In this lecture he emphasized that the scientific physician should address the anatomy, pathology and physiology of each patient with neurological disease. He conceived of the nervous system as an aggregate of discrete organs, each with a single function. Analysing a single symptom, hemiplegia, he showed that it was possible to diagnose focal pathology in the central nervous system.

He began this lecture, which was published in the *Reports* of the London Hospital, with his first quotation from a non-medical source, Bacon's dictum, "It is easier to evolve truth from error than from confusion."[40] He said that most physicians believed that the major impediment to understanding neurological diseases is the lack of a method for doing so. In proposing his method, he claimed that his was a natural rather than an artificial system. His procedure was aimed to be practical, and he recommended that those who did not find it useful should simply abandon it.

---

[37] J Hughlings Jackson, *Suggestions for studying diseases of the nervous system on Professor Owen's vertebral theory*, London, H K Lewis, 1863, on p. 1.
[38] Ibid., on p. iv.
[39] Hughlings Jackson, 'On the study of diseases of the nervous system', op. cit., note 21 above.
[40] Ibid., on p. 146.

Introduction

Hughlings Jackson advocated an expressly biological approach to case study, adding an explicit consideration of physiology to every study. He wrote,

> Just as we study, as physiologists and anatomists, the vegetative life of general tissues, the structure of organs for special functions, and the universal harmony of most diverse functions in individuals, so we ought, as workers in the field of Practical Medicine, to study every case that comes before us; as presenting
>
> 1. DISEASE OF TISSUE. (Changes in tissue)
> 2. DAMAGE OF ORGANS.
> 3. DISORDER OF FUNCTION.[41]

He expanded on this method with a consideration of rheumatic heart disease, noting that rheumatic fever was systemic, featuring focal disease in multiple organs including heart, liver and lung. Showing his wit, he gave his listeners a piece of advice. He told them never to treat patients on stethoscopic evidence only, since the heart may be a poor musical instrument but a good pump. He likened treating on stethoscopic evidence alone to a drunken ship's captain who navigated his ship around a speck of dirt on his chart, mistaking it for an island.[42]

He then turned his technique to diseases of the nervous system. He pointed out that the physiology of diseases of the optic, facial and ulnar nerves is very different, with dramatically different symptoms, yet their pathology might be similar.[43] He observed that diseases of the nervous system are not necessarily diseases of nervous tissue. For example, pathology of the vascular system or of connective tissue may disorder nervous function.

Hughlings Jackson insisted that knowing the exact organ or organs of the nervous system affected is crucially important for accurate diagnosis. He illustrated this dictum with the observation that hemiplegia may be seen in cortical syphilis, middle cerebral artery embolism, striatal haemorrhage or striatal tumour. In other words, a single symptom, hemiplegia, in a single organ, the corpus striatum, may be caused by four different pathologies.[44] He also pointed out that hemiplegia can occur with diseases in different anatomical locations, namely the striatum, crus cerebri, pons and medulla.[45] Hence, at the bedside, the physician cannot diagnose the cause of hemiplegia without considering its localization.

Hughlings Jackson's lecture elicited some note in the metropolis, being mentioned in the *British Medical Journal*.[46] More importantly, it gave him a reliable method for studying neurological disease, a method that he was soon to employ to dramatic effect. His first foray into theoretical neurology, which consisted mainly of the exposition of a system of study, was enough to give him a measure of notoriety in the capital. His next publication, a collection of patients with rheumatic heart disease, left middle cerebral artery embolism, right hemiparesis and aphasia, would thrust him into the centre of the dominant debate of nineteenth-century neurophysiology: what, exactly, are the functions of the nervous system?

---

[41] Ibid., on p. 147.
[42] Ibid., p. 149.
[43] Ibid., p. 152.
[44] Ibid., pp. 157–158.
[45] ibid., p. 157.
[46] 'Clinical lectures and reports by the medical and surgical staff of the London Hospital', *Br Med J*, 1864, **ii**: 523–524, p. 524.

Introduction

The Nature of the Epileptic Discharge

Hughlings Jackson's first recorded neurological writing appears in the 5 February 1859 entry of the Minute Book of the York Medical Society.[47] In a discussion of facial palsy, he quoted Todd in support of his views. Todd had written, "The phenomena of the epileptic fit depend upon a disturbed state of the nervous force, in certain parts of the brain—a morbidly excited polarity."[48] Influenced by his friend Michael Faraday, Todd conceived of nervous force as an electrical force.[49] He taught that paralysis and spasm of muscles are reciprocal events occurring in the same location in the brain.[50] Hughlings Jackson referred often to Todd's published clinical lectures, and he adopted the analytical principle that focal necrosis and focal seizures are physiologically reciprocal processes.

In an 1866 note on ocular deviation in epilepsy, Hughlings Jackson wrote that in unilateral convulsions the corpus striatum was stimulated.[51] In saying this he disagreed with the prevailing view that epilepsy was due to suppression rather than excitation of function. Convinced, like Todd, that hemiplegia and unilateral convulsions were in some way reciprocal, and that disease of the same nervous tissue could lead to either epilepsy or paralysis, he had to find a more physiologically detailed version of Todd's morbidly excited polarity.

In an 1867 paper comparing regional palsy and spasm, Hughlings Jackson described epilepsy as a "sudden disorderly expenditure of force".[52] Later that year he expanded this view to assert that epilepsy occurs when "the ill-nourished nerve-tissue is more unstable, over-ready, 'excitable;' there is discharge too soon; its Time is shortened."[53] In his 1869 Goulstonian lectures, Hughlings Jackson again contrasted the depletion of nervous force in hemiplegia with the disorderly discharge of stored force in unilateral convulsion.[54]

Shortly thereafter Hughlings Jackson published 'A study of convulsions' in the 1869 *Transactions* of the St Andrews Medical Graduates' Association, printed in 1870. This neurological classic begins with the observation that "a convulsion is but a symptom, and implies only that there is an occasional, an excessive, and a disorderly discharge of nerve tissue on muscles".[55] In this classical description of the epileptic discharge, Hughlings Jackson assumed that the epileptic discharge originated in the cortex, notwithstanding the conventional belief that the cortex was inexcitable. He let stand the possibility that the

---

[47] Greenblatt, op. cit., note 3 above, p. 350.

[48] Robert Bentley Todd, *Clinical lectures on paralysis, diseases of the brain, and other affections of the nervous system*, Philadelphia, Lindsay and Blakiston, 1855, p. 204.

[49] Edward H Reynolds, 'Todd, Faraday and the electrical basis of epilepsy', *Epilepsia*, 2004, **45**: 985–992.

[50] Todd, op. cit., note 48 above, pp. 204–205.

[51] J Hughlings Jackson, 'Note on lateral deviation of the eyes in hemiplegia and in certain epileptiform seizures', *Lancet*, 1866, **i**: 311–312, p. 311.

[52] J Hughlings Jackson, 'Note on the comparison and contrast of regional palsy and spasm', *Lancet*, 1867, **i**: 295–297, p. 296.

[53] J Hughlings Jackson, 'Remarks on the disorderly movements of chorea and convulsion', *Med Times Gaz*, 1867, **ii**: 642–643, p. 643.

[54] J Hughlings Jackson, 'Abstract of the Gulstonian [*sic*] lectures on certain points in the study and classification of diseases of the nervous system. Delivered at the Royal College of Physicians', *Lancet*, 1869, **i**: 307–308.

[55] J Hughlings Jackson, 'A study of convulsions', op. cit., note 27 above, p. 162.

epileptic discharge depends on instability of grey matter in either the cortex or the striatum. This uncertainty was resolved by Fritsch and Hitzig's 1870 demonstration that direct electrical stimulation of different parts of the cortex in dogs evoked movement of different parts of the body. These results led Hughlings Jackson to his 1873 dictum on the nature of the epileptic discharge: "Epilepsy is the name for occasional, sudden, excessive, rapid, and local discharge of grey matter."[56]

Some commentators describe Hughlings Jackson's principle of the discharge of nervous force as an electrical theory, and credit him with the first electrical theory of epilepsy.[57] However, he never employed the terminology of electricity or polarity in describing epilepsy. Hutchinson tells us that chemistry was his first love, dating to his days at York Medical School.[58] He had a chemical orientation to brain function, and his conception of the epileptic discharge was chemical, not electrical.

In the first of his 1890 Lumleian lectures on epilepsy, Hughlings Jackson defined nervous discharge as the liberation of energy by nervous elements.[59] Accepting that nervous discharges occur in health, he described the epileptic discharge as sudden, temporary and excessive in nature, a kind of explosive discharge. In his second Lumleian lecture he used a chemical analysis to describe the epileptic discharge, saying that it is a "physiological fulminate" like the gunpowder in a cannon.[60] Just as gunpowder can store energy that is liberated when the gun is fired, so the energy stored in nerve cells can be explosively liberated in an epileptic discharge. He never mentions batteries, current or any other electrical ideas. Hence his theory must be considered a chemical theory rather than an electrical one.

Jacksonian Epilepsy

Somatotopic representation, the principle that different parts of the nervous system represent the sensation and movement of different body parts, is a cornerstone of diagnostic neurology. Physicians use the distribution of a patient's weakness or sensory loss to localize strokes and brain tumours. Yet this principle ran contrary to accepted physiology in 1860. At the time, experimental physiologists followed Pierre Flourens in believing that all parts of the cortex and striatum, indeed the entire brain, are equipotential. Citing avian studies, Flourens wrote that when one neurological faculty disappears they all disappear, when one sensation reoccurs they all reoccur, and when one faculty reappears, they all reappear.[61] He believed that all of the intellectual faculties reside in the brain, but are not further localized there. This physiology had the philosophical aim of demonstrating the

---

[56] J Hughlings Jackson, 'On the anatomical, physiological, and pathological investigations of epilepsies', *West Riding Lunatic Asylum Medical Reports*, 1873, **3**: 315–349.
[57] E H Reynolds, 'Todd, Hughlings Jackson, and the electrical basis of epilepsy', *Lancet*, 2001, **358**: 575–577.
[58] Jonathan Hutchinson, op. cit., note 19 above, p. 1553.
[59] J Hughlings Jackson, 'The Lumleian Lectures on convulsive seizures' *Lancet*, 1890, **i**: 685–688, p. 685.
[60] J Hughlings Jackson, 'The Lumleian Lectures on convulsive seizures', *Lancet*, 1890, **i**: 735–738, p. 736.
[61] Pierre Flourens, *Recherches expérimentales sur les propriétés et les fonctions du système nerveux, dans les animaux vertébrés*, Paris, Crevot, 1824. Translated as 'Investigations of the properties and the functions of the various parts which compose the cerebral mass', in Gerhardt von Bonin (trans.), *Some papers on the cerebral cortex*, Springfield, ILL, Charles C Thomas, 1960, pp. 3–21.

truth of Cartesian dualism. Flourens believed that the metaphysical soul resides in the brain, and that the soul was elemental and hence indivisible. If the soul is indivisible, then the brain must be similarly indivisible.[62]

Physicians approached the problem differently. In 1835, Richard Bright described a patient who was admitted to Guy's Hospital following a series of right-sided convulsions. Between attacks he had transient right hemiparesis. While hospitalized, the patient had a right-sided convulsion, during which he remained conscious. Bright wrote, "These fits were owing to some local disorganization affecting the membranes and cineritious portion of the brain on the left side, and probably influencing the deep seated parts about the posterior end of the corpus striatum."[63]

At post-mortem, the patient had a subdural empyema over the left hemisphere. Bright used this case to illustrate that the left side of the striatum controlled the movement of the right side of the body. The phenomenon of lateralization, which was well known to physicians and surgeons, cast doubt on Flourens's idea of the equipotentiality of the nervous system, but was based on clinical examination rather than experimentation.

Hughlings Jackson described a common clinical occurrence which convincingly demonstrates somatotopic representation of movements in the nervous system. In some people, myoclonic movements begin in a restricted part of the body, commonly the hand, and march through one side of the body. Assuming that epileptic discharges spread from one part of the brain to the other with time, Hughlings Jackson concluded that these seizures can mean only that different parts of the nervous system control different parts of the body. The eponym "Jacksonian seizures" has been attached to focal seizures that march through different parts of the body.

The work for which Hughlings Jackson's name is eponymized was published between December 1867 and December 1868. In the 21 December 1867 edition of the *Medical Times and Gazette* he wrote, "Then in unilateral convulsions the 'aura' nearly always begins in the hand; sometimes, however, in the side of the face, and rarely in the leg".[64] In other words, the fact that an aura may be felt first in different parts of the body means that the epileptic discharge may begin in different parts of the nervous system.

In an August 1868 commentary on the physiology and pathology of the nervous system, Hughlings Jackson wrote, "One of the most important questions we can ask an epileptic patient is, 'How does the fit begin?' "[65] He published his description and interpretation of the Jacksonian march on 19 December 1868.

> I think the mode of beginning makes a great difference as to the march of the fit. When the fit begins in the face, the convulsion in involving the arm may *go down* the limb ... When the

---

[62] Robert M Young, *Mind, brain and adaptation in the nineteenth century* (Oxford, Clarendon, 1970), reprinted Oxford, Oxford University Press, 1990, pp. 70–72.

[63] Richard Bright, 'Cases illustrative of the effects produced when the arteries and brain are diseased', *Guy's Hospital Reports*, 1836, **1**: 9–40, on p. 36.

[64] J Hughlings Jackson, 'Remarks on the disorderly movements of chorea and convulsion, and on localisation', *Med Times Gaz*, 1867, **ii**: 669–670, p. 669.

[65] J Hughlings Jackson, 'Notes on the physiology and pathology of the nervous system', *Med Times Gaz*, 1868, **ii**: 177–179, p. 178.

Introduction

fit begins in the leg, the convulsion marches up; when the leg is affected after the arm, the convulsion marches *down* the leg.[66] [Emphasis in the original]

The importance of the Jacksonian march to clinical neurophysiology lies in its demonstration of somatotopic representation of the body in the nervous system. The march of ictal movements through the body recapitulates the order of anatomical representation of parts of the body in both the corpus striatum and the cortex. The Jacksonian march disproved the theory that all parts of the nervous system are functionally equipotential and validated the clinical concept that analysis of the temporal development of a focal neurological deficit is diagnostically useful. The knowledge of somatotopic representation allowed the astute neurologist to predict accurately the presence of focal pathology in the nervous system.

Jean-Martin Charcot first used the eponym "Jacksonian epilepsy". He noted that Louis-François Bravais had described the phenomenon in 1827, a priority which Hughlings Jackson accepted.[67] Charcot wrote:

> ... but lately, an English scholar, Mr. Jackson of London, came back to this subject, and he discussed the issue in a way so particular that it sometimes occurred to me to call that disorder Jacksonian epilepsy and the name remained associated ever since ... Mr. Jackson's study is so important that he really deserves his name to remain connected with this discovery.[68]

Charcot proposed to use the eponym "Bravais–Jackson" as an alternative: "it would be fairer; it is true that it would be somewhat long", but posterity has settled on the eponym "Jacksonian epilepsy". Charcot recognized the clinical utility of the principle of somatotopic representation, a crucial diagnostic tool for the astute neurologist.

Cerebral Localization

Hughlings Jackson produced a simple, flexible scheme of cerebral localization based on evolutionary neurophysiology that is the foundation of bedside diagnosis and modern neuroscience more generally. His scheme had four components. First, the nervous system is a sensorimotor machine. Second, somatotopic representation is a weighted, ordinal process. Third, the nervous system is a hierarchy of evolutionary levels, with higher levels suppressing the function of lower ones. Fourth, the nervous system and the mind exist in parallel, neither exerting a causal effect on the other. When combined at the bedside, these principles can allow the clever examiner to predict accurately the presence of pathology in the nervous system.

---

[66] J Hughlings Jackson, 'Notes on the physiology and pathology of the nervous system', *Med Times Gaz*, 1868, **ii**: 696.

[67] L-F Bravais, *Recherches sur les symptômes et le traitement de l'épilepsie hémiplégique*, Paris, Didot le Jeune, 1827 (thèse de Paris, no. 118).

[68] Jean-Martin Charcot, *Leçons du mardi à la Salpêtrière*, Paris, Delahaye & Lecrosnier, 1887, p.15: "Mais dans ces derniers temps, un savant anglais, M. Jackson (de Londres), est revenu sur ce sujet et il a traité la question d'une façon si particulière qu'il m'est arrivé quelquefois d'appeler cette affection l'épilepsie Jacksonienne et le nom lui en est resté.... l'étude de M. Jackson est si importante que véritablement, il méritait bien d'attacher son nom à cette découverte." And "ce serait plus juste; il est vrai que ce serait un peu long".

Introduction

The Sensorimotor Machine

In 1811, Charles Bell published a privately circulated book in which he described an experiment in anaesthetized dogs. When he pricked the anterior spinal root he produced movement, but when he pricked the posterior root he produced no movement. He concluded that the anterior root was responsible for movement.[69] In 1822, François Magendie divided the anterior root in dogs and produced paralysis, and divided the posterior root and produced anaesthesia. He concluded that the two roots were responsible for different functions, the anterior root being motor and the posterior root sensory.[70] This became known as the Bell–Magendie hypothesis or law, which is the source of a vigorous and unresolved dispute over priority of discovery.

In 1832, the English physiologist Marshall Hall reported an experiment in which stimulation of the limbs of a decapitated turtle produced reflex movement; if the spinal cord was destroyed this reflex movement was abolished.[71] Hall thus demonstrated that an intact spinal segment was necessary for reflex movement, with no need for supra-segmental influence. In a paper read to the Zoological Society, he was reported to have said that "the presence of the spinal marrow is essential as the central and cementing link between the sentient and motor nerves".[72] This led Hall to promulgate a physiological principle, known as the "law of reflex action", that stated that the behaviour of the isolated spinal segment could be completely explained by the action of reflexes.

Thomas Laycock wrote on the reflex action of the nervous system, beginning in 1840. In a paper read before the Medical Section of the British Association for the Advancement of Science in 1844, he proposed the general principle that the entire brain must be subject to the law of reflex action, since it is anatomically continuous with the spinal cord.[73] This implied that no metaphysical agent was necessary to explain the function of the nervous system. Laycock was later to teach Hughlings Jackson the principles and practice of medicine at York Medical School, and heavily influenced the younger man's neurophysiological thinking.[74] Hughlings Jackson quoted Laycock's paper several times in support of his contention that the nervous system is a sensorimotor machine.

The place of the metaphysical in the action of the nervous system hindered progress in neurophysiology in the mid-nineteenth century. Those who propounded ideas of sensation or movement without invoking the metaphysical properties of the soul were at risk of personal and professional criticism on theological grounds. Nevertheless, Hughlings Jackson made the claim that the action of the nervous system was not only sensorimotor, it was exclusively so.

---

[69] Charles Bell, *Idea for a new anatomy of the brain; submitted for the observations of his friends*, printed for private circulation, London, Strahan and Preston, 1811. Reprinted in facsimile in Paul F Cranefield (ed.), *The way in and the way out*, New York, Futura, 1974. The facsimile retains the pagination of the original pamphlet.

[70] François Magendie, 'Expériences sur les fonctions des racines des nerfs rachidiens', *Journal de physiologie expérimentale et pathologique*, 1822, **2**: 276–279. Reprinted in facsimile in Paul F Cranefield, *The way in and the way out*, New York, Futura, 1974. The facsimile retains the pagination of the original article.

[71] Marshall Hall, *Memoirs on the nervous system*, London, Sherwood, Gilbert and Piper, 1837, p. vi.

[72] Ibid., p. vi.

[73] T Laycock, 'On the reflex function of the brain', *Br Foreign Med Rev*, 1845, **19**: 298–311.

[74] Greenblatt, op. cit., note 3 above, pp. 348–349.

Introduction

As early as 1864, Hughlings Jackson referred obliquely to Laycock's application of the law of reflex action to the brain, though he did not elaborate on it.[75] In his 1870 'Study of convulsions' he concluded that some part of the cortex had sensorimotor function, writing "Are we to believe that the hemisphere is built on a plan *fundamentally* different from that of the motor tract?"[76] By 1874 he claimed that the nervous system is exclusively sensorimotor, writing, "The whole of the central nervous system, cerebral hemisphere, spinal cord, &c., is made up of processes of differing degrees of complexity representing impressions and movements. There are, so far as I can judge, no other 'materials' of which the 'organ of mind' can be made up."[77] He stated this principle more succinctly in 1883 when he wrote, "The whole nervous system is a sensori-motor machine, a co-ordinating system from top to bottom."[78] In 1887 he justified this opinion by reference to the law of conservation of energy, saying that immaterial agents such as volition, ideas and emotion cannot cause movement.[79]

This treatment of the nervous system as a machine, a soulless automaton, had both practical and personal origins. Hughlings Jackson was a committed physician, whose primary goal was to establish a workable system of diagnosis. A mechanical approach to neurophysiology proved powerfully heuristic. Moreover, Hughlings Jackson was a lifelong agnostic and strongly opposed metaphysical explanations of natural phenomena.[80] There is no record of Hughlings Jackson having suffered any public sanction for promoting his ostensibly atheistic physiological doctrine; whether he was privately criticized is not known.

Weighted Ordinal Representation

Hughlings Jackson, following in the footsteps of Todd, considered focal seizures in a limb and paralysis of the same limb as reciprocal events occurring in the same part of the nervous system. This way of thinking presented him with an apparent contradiction. As he pointed out in a December 1867 note on localization, patients with mild hemiparesis have slight weakness on an entire limb rather than severe weakness of a single muscle or movement. He took this to mean that each movement is represented in every part of the motor system, a holistic type of physiology. At the same time, the march of myoclonic movements through a limb in a Jacksonian seizure implies that each part is represented in a discrete part, a localizing type of physiology. To resolve these apparently contradictory physiological conceptions, Hughlings Jackson wrote, "So the speculation is that, although each movement is everywhere represented, there are points where particular movements are specially represented."[81]

---

[75] Hughlings Jackson, 'Loss of speech', op. cit., note 21 above, p. 454.
[76] Hughlings Jackson, op. cit., note 27 above, p. 189n.
[77] Hughlings Jackson, op. cit., note 29 above, 1874, **18**: 347–352, on p. 348.
[78] J Hughlings Jackson, 'On some implications of dissolution of the nervous system', *Med Press Circular*, 1883, **36**: 64–66, on p. 66.
[79] J Hughlings Jackson, 'Remarks on evolution and dissolution of the nervous system', *J Mental Sci.*, 1887, **33**: 25–48, on p. 40.
[80] Jonathan Hutchinson, op. cit., note 19 above, pp. 1551–1554, p. 1553.
[81] Hughlings Jackson, op. cit., note 64 above, page 669.

Introduction

Table 1
A graphical depiction of weighted representation. F stands for the face, A for the arm,
L for the leg. Weighting is depicted in bold characters

FAL	F**A**L	FA**L**

Special or weighted representation of body parts in a fundamentally holistic anatomical centre is graphically depicted in Table 1. In this depiction, each centre contains a complete representation of the body, but each centre is weighted for a different body part. Necrosis of a single centre causes some weakness of the entire body, but much more weakness in the specific body part specially represented in that centre. An epileptic discharge beginning in one centre and moving to the contiguous ones causes a march of myoclonic movements.

Conventional neurophysiology in 1860 asserted that the will or the metaphysical soul controls or regulates the function of the cortex, which in turn controls the rest of the nervous system. Hughlings Jackson accepted the idea of control of function but rejected an immaterial agent of control. Rather, he conceived of a hierarchy of sensorimotor centres in which anatomically higher centres control the function of lower centres. He saw the nervous system as a three-level hierarchy which he called lower, middle and highest centres. He further asserted that each element of the middle and highest centres contains a complete representation of the next lower level.

Table 2
A graphical depiction of weighted ordinal representation. F stands for the face, A for the arm, L for the leg. Middle level weighting is depicted in bold characters, highest level weighting is depicted by underlined characters

Highest level	<u>F</u>AL FAL FAL	F<u>A</u>L F<u>**A**</u>L F**A**L	FA<u>L</u> FAL F<u>**A**</u>**L**
Middle level	**F**AL	F**A**L	FA**L**
Lowest level	Face	Arm	Leg

The three-level hierarchy is graphically depicted in Table 2. In this depiction, each centre in the middle and highest levels contains a complete representation of the next lower level, but each is also weighted for a particular body part.

This scheme explains the partial weakness of an entire limb in mild hemiparesis because each centre in the middle level and highest levels contains a full representation of the body, and loss of it causes weakness throughout the body. It also explains the march of movements in a Jacksonian seizure because each centre is weighted for a different body part. This type of nested representation is ordinal, in the sense that each level is ordered by inclusion.

Introduction

Evolutionary Neurophysiology

The scientific and cultural firestorm that followed the publication of *On the origin of species* extended to medicine, leading Hughlings Jackson to apply explicitly evolutionary principles to neurophysiology. In his series of articles on the investigation of epilepsy, printed in the weekly *Medical Press and Circular* from 1874 to 1876, Hughlings Jackson adapted Herbert Spencer's evolutionary theory to neurological disease. In this series of articles he addressed the relationship between the centres in his hierarchy, concluding that this relationship conformed to evolutionary principles. Following Spencer, he concluded that the highest nervous centres evolved out of the lower. He wrote, "The very highest of all nervous centres are but complex rearrangements of lower centres, and these of still lower centres unto the lowest, which last *directly* represent impression and movements."[82] In 1882 he stated, "The higher the centre the more numerous, different, and more complex, and more special movements it represents."[83]

Hughlings Jackson expressed the pathophysiology of the nervous system as the reverse of evolution, or dissolution. As early as 1873 he asserted that patients with dissolution of the nervous system should exhibit symptoms which are less evolved than usual. He interpreted this to mean that a patient's symptoms should be less complex, less specialized and less voluntary than normal subjects.[84] Patients with diseases of the highest centres develop two types of symptoms, negative symptoms due to the loss of higher centres and positive symptoms due to the emergence of lower centres. Positive symptoms are simpler and less differentiated than the negative symptoms which they replace.

In 1875, Hughlings Jackson used post-ictal mental disorders to illustrate the relationship of the cortex to the basal ganglia.[85] If the sudden discharge of nervous energy produces an epileptic seizure, then seizures which begin with discharge of higher centres start with loss of consciousness, but those which begin with discharge of lower centres spare consciousness. According to Hughlings Jackson, post-ictal mental symptoms, like post-ictal physical ones, have the two components predicted by evolutionary theory: the negative symptom of post-ictal confusion, from the temporary paralysis of higher centres, and the positive symptoms of post-ictal mania or agitation, from the emergence of the function of the previously inhibited lower centres.

Over the succeeding years Hughlings Jackson elaborated these themes. In 1882 he identified the specific anatomic structures corresponding to each motor level. The lowest level, representing parts of the body most directly, consists of the anterior spinal horns and homologous cranial motor nerve nuclei. The middle level, which re-represents the body, is composed of the motor cortex and the basal ganglia. The highest level, which re-re-represents the body, consists of the premotor frontal cortex.[86]

---

[82] Hughlings Jackson, op. cit., note 29 above, 1874, **18**: 347–352, on p. 348.

[83] J Hughlings Jackson, 'On some implications of dissolution of the nervous system', *Med Press Circular*, 1882, **34**: 411–414, on p. 412.

[84] J Hughlings Jackson, 'On the anatomical and physiological localisation of movements in the brain', *Lancet*, 1873, **i**: 84–85.

[85] J Hughlings Jackson, 'On temporary mental disorders after epileptic paroxysms', *West Riding Lunatic Asylum Medical Reports*, 1875, **5**: 105–129.

[86] Hughlings Jackson, op. cit., note 83 above.

Introduction

In his March 1884 Croonian lectures, Hughlings Jackson presented his mature theory of cerebral localization as practical evolutionary physiology. Delivered at the Royal College of Physicians in London, these lectures were published in the *British Medical Journal*, the *Lancet*, and the *Medical Times and Gazette*. In them, Hughlings Jackson presented to the world a detailed explication of his evolutionary neurophysiology.[87] In his first lecture he reiterated the dual nature of neurological symptoms. He claimed that, "the symptomatology of nervous diseases is a double condition; there is a negative and a positive element in every case".[88]

He went on to point out that disease or dissolution can be uniformly distributed through the nervous system or can be confined to a small local area. Focal dissolution can involve one neurological system or several, and could extend through one or two evolutionary levels. He wrote,

> We make two broad divisions of cases of dissolution, Uniform and Local. In Uniform Dissolution the whole of the nervous system is under the same conditions or evil influence; the evolution of the whole nervous system is comparatively evenly reversed ... The next division is Local Dissolution. Obviously, disease of a part of the nervous system could not be a reversal of the evolution of the whole; all that we can expect is a local reversal of evolution ...[89]

In his second lecture Hughlings Jackson introduced the idea of tonic inhibition, set in evolutionary terms. He claimed that higher levels suppress the function of lower levels:

> The higher nervous arrangements evolved out of the lower keep down those lower, just as a government evolved out of a nation controls as well as directs that nation. If this be the process of evolution, then the reverse process of dissolution is not only a "taking off" of the higher, but is at the very same time a "letting go" of the lower.[90]

The Doctrine of Concomitance

In his third Croonian lecture Hughlings Jackson first enunciated his doctrine of concomitance. He asserted that the nervous system is an explicitly sensorimotor machine arranged as an evolutionary hierarchy. He recognized human consciousness as the highest level of mental evolution, the analogue of the highest level of evolution of the nervous system. This generated an urgent question: how, if at all, are these two highest expressions of evolution related to one another?

Hughlings Jackson knew at least three theoretical solutions to the mind–body problem. In the first, the "mind acts through the nervous system ... here an immaterial agency is supposed to produce physical effects".[91] Though he does not mention Descartes, this

---

[87] Hughlings Jackson, op. cit., note 31 above. See also J Hughlings Jackson, 'Croonian lectures on the evolution and dissolution of the nervous system. Delivered at the Royal College of Physicians', *Lancet*, 1884, **i**: 555–558, 649–652, 739–744, and J Hughlings Jackson, 'Croonian lectures on evolution and dissolution of the nervous system. Delivered at the Royal College of Physicians', *Med Times Gaz*, 1884, **i**: 411–413, 445–448, 649–652. The published lectures were, in part, transcribed verbatim by an unknown note-taker, and in part paraphrased.
[88] Hughlings Jackson, op. cit., note 31 above, p. 591.
[89] Ibid., p. 591.
[90] Ibid., p. 662.
[91] Hughlings Jackson, op. cit., note 79 above, p. 37.

Introduction

version can be recognized as Cartesian dualism. In the second solution, "activities of the highest centres and mental states are one and the same thing",[92] a statement of the mind–brain identity theory. The third version says that brain states and mental states are intrinsically different, occur in parallel and have no causal interaction between them.[93] This brain–mind theory, a form of psychophysical parallelism, Hughlings Jackson called the doctrine of concomitance.

Hughlings Jackson recognized that any solution to the mind–body problem was not a medical but a philosophical theory, which he specifically termed metaphysical. Under most circumstances he strongly rejected metaphysical explanations for medical observations, even denying that comatose persons were unconscious, because consciousness is a metaphysical concept. None the less, he embraced the doctrine of concomitance because it allowed a practical analysis of neurological disease which conformed to his clinical observation.[94]

The doctrine of concomitance was not Hughlings Jackson's invention. He claimed that a number of other Victorian scientists and philosophers held similar views, including Thomas Henry Huxley, John Stuart Mill, Alexander Bain, Herbert Spencer and Thomas Laycock.[95] The basic idea can be traced to the work of the German philosopher Leibniz, which was known to both Laycock and Hughlings Jackson.[96] The latter admitted that his doctrine of concomitance could be construed as a form of Leibniz's "two clock theory", in which one clock is timed to strike when the other showed the hour.[97] This is taken as an analogy of the non-causal parallelism of brain and mind.

The Rejection of the Unconscious

Hughlings Jackson's assertion that the mind exists in parallel to the nervous system, and that the nervous system has an evolutionary structure, led him to subject the mind to a similar evolutionary analysis. Consciousness, as the highest level of mental evolution, could be seen as the most complex, most specialized, most integrated, and most interconnected mental function, analogous to the highest level of the nervous system.[98] As a practical physician, he sought to find evolutionary levels of the mind, with the aim to treat mental disease.

Hughlings Jackson reasoned that the structure of the mind should strictly follow the structure of the nervous system. He thought that if the nervous system is composed of evolutionary levels connected by a process of representation, and if the mind and the brain are related by the doctrine of concomitance, then the mind can also be understood as having evolutionary levels connected by representation. Furthermore, just as states of the highest

---

[92] Ibid.
[93] Ibid.
[94] Ibid., pp. 38–39.
[95] Ibid., p. 38.
[96] Ibid. See also Thomas Laycock, *Mind and brain: or, the correlations of consciousness and organization, with their applications to philosophy, zoology, physiology, mental pathology, and the practice of medicine*, Edinburgh, Sutherland and Knox, 1860, p. 183. Laycock comments, "In Germany, the doctrine of Leibniz was almost universally adopted."
[97] Hughlings Jackson, op. cit., note 79 above, p. 38.
[98] Ibid., p. 39.

Introduction

level of nervous evolution have concomitant mental states, so states of the middle and lower levels of nervous evolution should have concomitant mental levels. It stands to reason that any mental state lower than consciousness is unconscious. Hence, if the combination of nervous system evolution and concomitance is correct, then unconscious mental states must exist as the logical concomitants of lower levels of evolution of the nervous system. This brought Hughlings Jackson to consider the following question: how far down the evolutionary hierarchy of the nervous system are there concomitant mental states? In Hughlings Jackson's words, "What is the range of concomitance?"[99]

Even before he enunciated his doctrine of concomitance, he accepted the existence of unconscious mental states and actions as the source of spoken words. In an 1878 article on aphasia, published in the first volume of the journal *Brain*, he wrote that "perception is the termination of a stage beginning by the unconscious or subconscious revival of images".[100] Echoing the ideas of G H Lewes, he noted the possibility that all nervous centres have a psychological side, presumably including the spinal cord.[101]

Four years later he expressed more serious reservations about the existence of unconscious mental states. In an 1881 series of articles on post-epileptic states he claimed that all mental states have concomitant physical states, but asked the question whether the converse is true.[102] Specifically, he asked whether states of the lower nervous centres have concomitant mental states. He wrote, "Is there any sort of subconsciousness or sensibility or any sort of psychical state, however rudimentary, attending functioning of any lower nervous arrangements? . . . I express no opinion on this most difficult question."[103] In his third Croonian lecture he again attributed to Lewes the thesis that some degree of consciousness attends activity of all levels of nervous activity. However, by this time he seemed inclined to deny that unconscious states of mind existed, though he again was unsure. He wrote, "Some, indeed, speak of 'unconscious states of mind,' as if, below consciousness, there were some faint mental states. I am not sure that I state this view with verbal correctness, as I do not understand it."[104]

In his April 1887 commentary on the evolution and dissolution of the nervous system he returned to a discussion of the range of concomitance.[105] He stated that he thought that the entire body is the organ of mind, but asks that, for the sake of argument, the highest level of the nervous system be considered the organ of mind. He then asserted that consciousness and mind are synonymous terms. Following this, he explicitly rejected unconscious mental states:

> Unconscious states of mind are sometimes spoken of, which seems to me to involve a contradiction. That there may be activities of lower nervous arrangements of the highest centres, which have no attendant psychical states, and which yet lead to next activities of the very highest nervous arrangements of those centres whose activities have attendant psychical

---

[99] Ibid., p. 39.

[100] J Hughlings Jackson, 'On affections of speech from disease of the brain', *Brain*, 1878, **1**: 304–330, p. 325.

[101] Ibid., footnote on p. 323.

[102] J Hughlings Jackson, 'Remarks on dissolution of the nervous system, as exemplified by certain post-epileptic conditions', *Med Press Circular*, 1881, **31**: 329–332, 399–400, 1881, **32**: 68–70, 380–382, 399–401, 421–422.

[103] Ibid., **32**: 69.

[104] Hughlings Jackson, op. cit., note 31 above, p. 706.

[105] Hughlings Jackson, op. cit., note 79 above.

states, I can easily understand. But those prior activities are states of the nervous system, not any sort of states of mind.[106]

This article exposes Hughlings Jackson's dilemma. He had concluded that if the highest level of brain evolution has the concomitant mental state of human consciousness, then lower levels of brain evolution also must have concomitant, unconscious, mental states. But no such states are apparent clinically; an unconscious patient is simply unresponsive. Hughlings Jackson resolved this by rejecting the entire idea of the unconscious, stating that any state of mind is by definition conscious, and indeed cannot be otherwise. Unconscious mental states are, for Hughlings Jackson, a contradiction.

Hughlings Jackson's change of mind was the result of his evolutionary thinking. If the nervous system is composed of discrete evolutionary levels, and if higher levels control or suppress the action of lower levels, then disease which affects a given level will have two symptoms. One symptom, a negative one, is the result of loss of function of the higher, controlling level; the other symptom, a positive one, is the result of the appearance of function of the lower, previously inhibited level. Hughlings Jackson's application of this method to the study of epilepsy and aphasia had striking practical value.

As an example of this method, Hughlings Jackson considered the symptoms of aphasia. He observed that aphasic patients cannot speak grammatically, cannot write and have difficulty with pantomime. He identified these as the negative element of the disease, reflecting dissolution of the highest level of the nervous system. He also observed that these patients utter stereotypic words or phrases, which at times have a clear semantic content and at other times are apparently meaningless. These recurrent utterances he identified as the positive element of the illness, which is an expression of the release or dis-inhibition of the middle evolutionary level.[107]

Hughlings Jackson used the same reasoning to consider the mind. If consciousness is the highest level of mental evolution, and a patient loses consciousness as the negative element of the illness, then what remains must be the positive expression of lower, unconscious mental function. However, as an experienced and astute physician, he had examined many unconscious patients, and he knew that an unconscious individual did not manifest any easily identifiable mental function at all. Instead, the patient lies in bed, mute and uncomprehending. Such a person offers little evidence of unconscious speech or action, despite showing unequivocal evidence of positive signs of function of lower levels of the nervous system.[108]

He also used the example of complex post-epileptic behaviour. He had observed that after epileptic fits some patients act elaborately, in ways which seem to involve complex mental activities. Later the patient has no memory of the event. He commented, "To say that the patient had unconscious or latent states of mind does not, I think, help us."[109] In other words, during a time of temporary dissolution of the nervous system, he could observe no states of mind which could be construed as unequivocally unconscious.

---

[106] Ibid., pp. 39–40.
[107] Hughlings Jackson, op. cit., note 100 above.
[108] Hughlings Jackson, op. cit., note 31 above, p. 661.
[109] Hughlings Jackson, op. cit., note 79 above, p. 40.

Introduction

Hughlings Jackson had a practical motivation for his rejection of the unconscious. His commitment to the idea of the nervous system as a sensorimotor machine made him reject explanations of nervous system disease in psychological or philosophical terms. As a physician, he aimed to develop a system that was useful at the bedside. This produced an extreme empiricism, so that he could not accept a theory that had no visible examples in everyday neurological practice. He specifically disavowed any philosophical interest in the mind–body relationship, saying, "I am not competent to discuss the metaphysical question of the *nature* of the relationship of mind to nervous activities."[110] Elsewhere he stated, "As an Evolutionist I am not concerned with this question, and for medical purposes I do not care about it."[111] This ultimately led to his perplexity in the case of the range of concomitance.

Hughlings Jackson changed his mind because his strict personal standards required him to reject ideas which he could not validate, even if those ideas were his own. His colleagues and friends tell us of his intellectual honesty and personal rectitude. Hutchinson said that his "love of truthfulness was very strong".[112] His colleague Charles Mercier remarked on his "high standards of rectitude".[113] His student and collaborator James Risien Russell wrote, "No sordid motives influenced him in his life-work, which goes down to posterity as a monument of his greatness."[114] In a man of such intellectual integrity, it does not seem out of character that he should reject his own previously held opinion if he could no longer defend it.

In summary, Hughlings Jackson initially assumed that the structure of the mind is exactly analogous to the structure of the nervous system. Applying this analogy to neurological diseases, pathological states involving the loss of consciousness should be accompanied by positive mental symptoms caused by dis-inhibition of sub-conscious mental states. Hughlings Jackson recognized that there was a problem with his analysis when he did not observe the predicted mental states in unconscious patients. He could explain this by altering either his assumption about the structure of the mind or the doctrine of concomitance that predicted that structure. He followed the latter course, rejecting the general interpretation of concomitance and restricting the range of concomitance to the highest level of evolution of the nervous system. In doing so he rejected the existence of unconscious mental states.

Aphasia

In 1864, Hughlings Jackson published a series of cases aimed at illustrating his method of case analysis in pathological, anatomical and physiological terms.[115] In this series, published in the London Hospital *Reports*, he collected 34 cases of patients with cardiac valvular

---

[110] Ibid., p. 37.

[111] Hughlings Jackson, 'On post-epileptic states: a contribution to the comparative study of insanities', *J Mental Sci*, 1888, **34**: 349–365, on p. 350.

[112] Jonathan Hutchinson, op. cit., note 19 above, p. 1553.

[113] 'The late Dr. Hughlings Jackson. Recollections by Dr. Mercier', *Br Med J*, 1912, **i**: 85–86, on p. 85. Obituary, *Br Med J*, op. cit., note 20 above, p. 953.

[114] Obituary, *Br Med J*, op. cit., note 20 above, p. 953.

[115] Hughlings Jackson, 'Loss of speech', op. cit., note 21 above.

Introduction

disease, hemiplegia and loss of speech. Asserting that the cause of the neurological symptoms was embolism to the middle cerebral artery, he found that 31 patients had right hemiplegia. He claimed no novelty in these observations, crediting Paul Broca with developing the principle that disease of the third left frontal convolution led to loss of articulate language. He wrote, "M. Broca believes that disease of the left side of the brain only, produces loss of Language; and moreover, he locates the faculty of Articulate Language in a very limited part of that hemisphere. My observations tend to support the first hypothesis, and, in a general way, the second."[116] He also credited Brown-Séquard, a friend of Broca, with teaching him to distinguish between speech, articulation and voice.

Hughlings Jackson's chief contribution to the aphasia debate was his rejection of the principle that brain functions are psycho-physiological faculties. Broca had distinguished between a general faculty of language, a mental faculty manifested in all forms of expression including sign language and writing, and a faculty of articulate language, or speaking. Hughlings Jackson, in his 1864 series, found that all patients had defects of all modalities of expression, yet had disease in the distribution of the left middle cerebral artery. He also observed that, in order to distinguish between troubles of articulation and speech, it is useful to have the patient attempt to communicate by writing.

By 1866 Hughlings Jackson had concluded that, although Broca's aphasia resulted from disease of the left frontal lobe, the faculty of articulate language, as such, did not exist. He wrote, "I think, then, that the so-called 'faculty' of language has no existence, and that disease near the corpus striatum produces defect of expression (by words, writing, signs, etc.) to a great extent, because this is the way out from the hemisphere to the organs which the will can set in motion."[117] That is, aphasic patients have normal mental function, but cannot translate inner language to speech. He distinguished between intellectual and emotional speech; Broca's aphasia affects intellectual speech, but the remaining utterances of aphasics represent the residual emotional speech. In an 1866 letter to the editor of the *Medical Times and Gazette*, he also made the interesting observation of the coexistence of aphasia and left hemiparesis in a patient who lamented his paralysis because he was left handed.[118]

Both Broca and Hughlings Jackson believed that the association of aphasia and hemiplegia was due to the combined disease of the cortex and the corpus striatum. Orthodox neurophysiological opinion held that the cortex served mental operations while the striatum served motor function, and that the cortex was inexcitable. In changing these beliefs, Hughlings Jackson made his most durable contribution, the fundamental principle of diagnostic neurology: the concept of evolutionary neurophysiology applied to the bedside.

Recovery

Hughlings Jackson's analysis of evolution and dissolution of the nervous system had to explain a common event in clinical practice, namely that people often recover substantially

---

[116] Ibid, on p. 388.

[117] J Hughlings Jackson, 'Notes on the physiology and pathology of language. Remarks on those cases of disease of the nervous system in which defect of expression is the most striking symptom', *Med Times Gaz*, 1866, **i**: 659–662, p. 660.

[118] J Hughlings Jackson, 'Hemiplegia of the left side, with defect of speech', *Med Times Gaz*, 1866, **ii**: 210.

after focal necrosis of the nervous system, for example after a stroke. His system of weighted ordinal representation, taken as a static system, could not explain this progressive recovery because, if the representation of the affected movement is fixed, then the degree to which undamaged areas can compensate should also be fixed. However, this conflicted with the clinical observation that, as time progressed after a focal brain injury, the affected movement steadily improved. Because of this, Hughlings Jackson concluded that the weighting of representation had to be a dynamic process, which he called the Principle of Compensation.

In Jacksonian compensation, if one element is damaged, other elements with less weighted representation continue to act, in proportion to their initial weighting. This includes elements of the same evolutionary level, and also elements of different levels. If more elements are damaged, fewer undamaged areas remain, and the degree of loss of function is greater. In addition, damage to higher levels produces less severe symptoms than damage to lower levels, because higher levels contain more complex and interconnected representations of the damaged area and therefore compensate more fully in the event of brain injury.

The concept of weighted representation meant that this system could be a dynamic one. Re-weighting of representation in undamaged areas of the nervous system implies that, in progressive recovery, some areas will become more active and others less active than in the normal, undamaged brain. This aspect caused Hughlings Jackson to write that the loss of a particular movement is "largely compensated in time by greater activity" of the remaining areas.[119] As time passes, there appears "to be decided paralysis of X only, but slowly the other terms come to serve for moving the whole region more efficiently and what is called the paralysis of X diminishes".[120]

While Hughlings Jackson's examples of compensation were most often taken from the motor system, he intended that it apply to the entire nervous system, including the somatosensory and special sensory systems. In an 1876 analysis of post-ictal paralysis, he raised doubts that total deafness or total blindness could result from cortical injury, because undamaged sensory areas could partially compensate for the damaged areas.[121] However, in a footnote, he raised the possibility that symmetrical damage to the appropriate cortical areas might completely obliterate vision or hearing. Nevertheless, he wrote that "the Principle of Compensation, I suppose, hold[s] for all nervous centres".[122]

Hughlings Jackson reasoned that, if compensation applied to circumstances in which parts of the nervous system were destroyed, it should also apply to clinical states in which parts of the nervous system were stimulated, namely epilepsy. In "inverted compensation", the disordered movements in a tonic-clonic seizure are the result of simultaneous discharge of many elements with different representation, including heavily weighted and other, more lightly weighted, areas. Movements elicited in this way, the result of

---

[119] Hughlings Jackson, 'On some implications of dissolution of the nervous system', *Med Press Circular*, 1882, **34**: 433–434, on p. 433.

[120] Ibid., p. 434.

[121] J Hughlings Jackson, 'On epilepsies and on the after-effects of epileptic discharges (Todd and Robertson's hypothesis)', *West Riding Lunatic Asylum Medical Reports*, 1876, **6**: 266–309.

[122] Ibid., p. 290.

activity of all motor areas acting simultaneously, were not normal but rather distinctly abnormal.[123]

Ophthalmology in its Relation to General Medicine

Hughlings Jackson's first hospital appointment was to the Royal London Ophthalmic Hospital, commonly called the Moorfields Eye Hospital. He recognized the importance of ophthalmology in the study of neurological disease, and carefully examined and reported eye findings in his cases. He integrated ophthalmology into scientific neurology, in the process measurably improving the sensitivity of bedside diagnosis. In recognition of his contributions to ophthalmology, he was selected to give the 1877 Annual Oration to the Medical Society of London, and the 1885 Bowman Lecture and 1889 Presidential Address to the Ophthalmological Society of the United Kingdom. In each lecture he described important ophthalmological findings in neurological disease.[124]

His classic 1877 lecture, entitled 'Ophthalmology in its relation to general medicine', contains a wealth of neurological insight.[125] He stressed the importance of routine ophthalmoscopic examination, and said that vision must be corrected refractively before it could be analysed neurologically. As an example of systematic ophthalmoscopy, he pointed to the fact that patients with brain tumours could have bilateral papilledema, which he called optic neuritis, despite normal vision. This fact obliged the practical physician to examine every patient's eyes ophthalmoscopically. At the same time, the examiner can evaluate the retinal vessels as an indirect indication of the state of the cerebral circulation. This technique allowed Hughlings Jackson to perform one of his two published experiments. Applying ice to the back of the head while simultaneously examining the retinal vessels, he concluded that this manoeuvre did not alter the cerebral blood flow.[126]

In his 1877 lecture he noted that patients with ocular signs of syphilis and focal seizures most likely have neurosyphilis, that diphtheria causes a unique ciliary paralysis, and that patients with ophthalmoplegia often complain of vertigo. He asserted that there are centres for conjoint movements of the eyes, which can be damaged unilaterally with diseases in the frontal cortex or the brainstem. Quoting Charcot, he noted that hemispheric disease could produce hemianopsia. Ophthalmoscopic examination could reveal ocular emboli and the signs of Bright's disease.[127]

---

[123] Hughlings Jackson, op. cit., note 119 above.

[124] J Hughlings Jackson, 'An address on ophthalmology in its relation to general medicine', *Br Med J*, 1877, **i**: 575–577, 605–606, 672–674, 703–705, 804–805; J Hughlings Jackson, 'Ophthalmology and diseases of the nervous system, being the Bowman lecture, delivered Friday, November 13th, 1885, *Trans Ophthalmol Soc U.K.*, 1886, **6**: 1–22; J Hughlings Jackson, 'Presidential address, delivered at the first meeting of the session, October 17th, 1889', *Trans Ophthalmol Soc U.K.*, 1890, **10**: xliv–lix. See also Burton Chance, 'Short studies on the history of ophthalmology. III. Hughlings Jackson, the neurologic ophthalmologist, with a summary of his works', *Arch Ophthalmol*, 1937, **17**: 241–289.

[125] *Br Med J*, 1877, **i**: 575–577, 605–606, 672–674, 703–705, 804–805.

[126] J Hughlings Jackson, 'An experimental inquiry into the effect of the application of ice to the back of the neck on the retinal circulation', *Med Times Gaz*, 1863, **ii**: 90–91.

[127] Hughlings Jackson, *Br Med J*, op. cit., note 125 above, pp. 703–704.

Introduction

Hughlings Jackson's Philosophy

Modern writers see a philosophical motivation in Hughlings Jackson's neurophysiology, which they attribute to either a youthful intent to abandon medicine in pursuit of a career in academic philosophy, or a mature interest in formal philosophy. However, an examination of his early crisis of intention in the context of his background and his personality reveal it to be a literary ambition of a sort common in Victorian Britain, rather than a desire to be an academic philosopher. Later, when discussing his neurological work, Hughlings Jackson expressly and repeatedly disclaimed philosophical motivation. Instead, he claimed that the needs of practical medicine motivated his theoretical work.

The story of Hughlings Jackson's youthful crisis of intention is found only in Hutchinson's 1911 *British Medical Journal* obituary, written fifty years after the events described.[128] Hutchinson's entire description of this episode, published a week after his friend's death, is as follows:

> When Dr. Jackson and myself first made acquaintance he had been some two or three years in the profession, and, in the belief that it did not afford attractive scope for mental powers of which he was not unconscious, he was on the point of abandoning it, intending to engage in a literary life. From this I was successful in dissuading him, and for many years I plumed myself upon this as the most successful achievement of my long life. Of late, however, I have had my misgivings, and have doubted whether—great as had been the gain to medicine—it might not have been a yet greater gain to the world at large if Hughlings Jackson had been left to devote his mind to philosophy. There are others who are better skilled than myself to give an opinion on this head, but at some future time I may hope to be able to produce some details in illustration of his character which may go far to justify my misgivings.[129]

Eight weeks later Hutchinson wrote a longer memoir, but did not expand on Hughlings Jackson's literary or philosophical ambitions.[130]

The young Hughlings Jackson was undoubtedly ambitious, but the nature and direction of his ambition must be viewed in context. Lacking university education, he had no chance of an academic career, philosophical or otherwise. He came from yeoman stock, and his family seem to have been religious dissenters. Therefore, he had very little chance of gaining admission to what might be called a philosophy school or graduate programme, much less being appointed to an academic position in philosophy.

Practical considerations of money and family give a more plausible explanation of this episode. Hughlings Jackson's father Samuel became impoverished late in his life, and, in the same period, his three brothers emigrated and his sister died. He might have received some compensation as a houseman, but he probably received little support from his family. With his father in straitened circumstances and in failing health, it appears quite likely that he lived a threadbare existence. In the summer of 1859 he moved to London permanently, short of money but burning with ambition and well aware of his own intellectual powers. It was at this time that he had his crisis of intention.

At the age of twenty-four, with little money, he no doubt sought to use his intellect to make a living, and he probably considered medicine only one of several options. For

---

[128] 'Obituary', *Br Med J*, op. cit., note 20 above.
[129] Ibid., p. 952.
[130] Hutchinson, op. cit., note 19 above.

Introduction

example, he must have known something of the law, since one of his brothers was a lawyer. He also read voraciously, most notably Carlyle and Dickens. In thinking how a self-aware, medically sophisticated intellectual might support himself in 1859 London, Hughlings Jackson must have considered some type of writing for money. Hutchinson would have interpreted this as a "literary life". There is no evidence that he considered writing fiction, though there is no *a priori* reason to reject this possibility. More likely, though, he was thinking of non-fiction or journalism. It seems far-fetched to imagine the ambitious young Hughlings Jackson taking rooms in a university to study philosophy, even had he the background to do so.

Furthermore, grand scientific syntheses were becoming a social and publishing phenomenon in mid-Victorian Britain. The success of Robert Chambers's *Vestiges of the natural history of creation*, first published in 1844, emboldened Darwin and Spencer to publish their own synthetic works. These volumes had wide appeal among the increasingly literate and prosperous public, as reflected in their sales. None of these writers were academic scientists, though they might be called literary scientists or even literary philosophers. An ambition to write treatises of synthetic science, rather than to pursue a career in academic philosophy, seems a better explanation of Hughlings Jackson's goal of a "literary life".

In later life Hughlings Jackson was a prolific writer. Assessing any writer's motivation is a difficult task, a task made doubly difficult in Hughlings Jackson's case because he had his executor burn his personal papers after his death. Little autograph material remains other than his published works, but he did leave a number of published comments about his creative motivation. These show him to be a practical physician whose primary motivation was medical science rather than theory or philosophy. Moreover, he published exclusively in medical journals, lectured mainly to medical audiences and spent his days practising medicine. Therefore he could expect to have his work seen and criticized by his fellow physicians, but not necessarily by academic scientists or academic philosophers.

Hughlings Jackson specifically rejected metaphysics and materialism, two areas of Victorian philosophical inquiry. In a preface to his 1875 pamphlet on cerebral localization, he said that it is possible to practise medicine with any type of metaphysical beliefs, or none at all: "That along with excitations or discharges of nervous arrangements in the cerebrum, mental states occur, I, of course, admit; but how this is I do not inquire; indeed, so far as clinical medicine is concerned, I do not care."[131] The next year, in a paper on Todd's paralysis, he wrote that the aim of his mechanical view of the nervous system was to combat metaphysical neurophysiology. He discounted the philosophical idea that there exists a centre of the nervous system that acts as a metaphysical interpreter, standing outside sensory and motor function.[132]

In an address to the Section of Pathology at the August 1882 meeting of the British Medical Association in Worcester, Hughlings Jackson criticized metaphysical

---

[131] J Hughlings Jackson, *Clinical and physiological researches on the nervous system. No. 1. On the localisation of movements in the brain*, London, J and A Churchill, 1875, held in the Rockefeller Library, Institute of Neurology, University College London. This item, including the preface, also appears in James Taylor (ed.), *Selected writings of John Hughlings Jackson*, 2 vols, London, Hodder and Stoughton, 1931–32. Reprinted New York, Basic Books, 1958, vol. 1, p. 52.

[132] Hughlings Jackson, op. cit., note 121 above, pp. 306–308.

Introduction

explanations of disease. He stated, "It is rather difficult to define metaphysics. Some people call psychology metaphysics; some call anything very difficult and complex about mind and body metaphysics; some use it merely as a term of abuse."[133] As an example of metaphysical explanations of disease he used the proposition that aphasic patients have lost words but not the memory of words. He said that, on the contrary, the words we speak and the words we think are the same thing; if not, mental words would be insubstantial. According to the law of conservation of energy, insubstantial phenomena cannot produce speech in any manner. He also lamented that medical students are not taught metaphysics, so they could be less metaphysical in their professional life. Saying that metaphysical explanations of hysteria explain nothing, he asserted that scientific physicians must steer clear of metaphysics.[134]

Hughlings Jackson took a dim view of materialism. In his third Croonian lecture he specifically disclaimed materialism, citing as sources a litany of scientists and writers including William Hamilton, John Stuart Mill, Herbert Spencer, Friedrich Max Müller, Alexander Bain, Thomas Henry Huxley, Emil Du Bois-Reymond, Thomas Laycock, John Tyndall and David Ferrier.[135] These men, with whom Hughlings Jackson identified as scientific peers, include physicians and philosophers, professors and writers, and one or two figures who defy categorization.

In his April 1887 remarks on evolution and dissolution of the nervous system, he said that a critic of his Croonian lectures had accused him of fabricating the doctrine of concomitance in order to avoid the charge of materialism, and of appropriating Leibniz's "two-clock theory". He replied that this might be true but it does not matter, because Leibniz's philosophy is irrelevant to medicine. He added that evolutionists need not invoke supernatural agency to explain natural phenomena. He claimed that it is impossible to localize mental function because the nervous system is exclusively sensorimotor and reiterated his discussion of mind–body theories, saying that he could accept a mind–body identity theory if it meant that the nervous system has two functions, integration and thinking. Even if the mind–brain identity theory is right, the doctrine of concomitance as an artifice is still useful for physicians because it separates practical bedside diagnosis from non-localized psychological function. According to Hughlings Jackson, mental disease may be present but its nature excludes it from the purview of medical science.

The Bibliography of John Hughlings Jackson

The primary sources which contain Hughlings Jackson's writings are not widely held, and no published collection of his works exists. As an appendix to the published text of his 1903 Hughlings Jackson Lecture, Sir William Broadbent gave the only bibliography published during Hughlings Jackson's life.[136] In 1931, Hughlings Jackson's student, collaborator, colleague and biographer James Taylor published the two-volume *Selected*

---

[133] J Hughlings Jackson, 'An address delivered at the opening of the section of pathology, at the annual meeting of the British Medical Association in Worcester, August 1882', *Br Med J*, 1882, **ii**: 305–308, p. 308.

[134] Ibid., p. 308.

[135] Hughlings Jackson, op. cit., note 31 above, p. 706.

[136] William Broadbent, 'Hughlings Jackson as a pioneer in nervous physiology and pathology', *Brain*, 1903, **26**: 305–366, pp. 356–366.

Introduction

writings of John Hughlings Jackson in collaboration with Gordon Holmes and Francis Walshe.[137] The second volume of this set contains a bibliography which is more complete than Broadbent's. Careful study reveals that both Broadbent's and Taylor's bibliographies are incomplete and inaccurate. In his classic work on the early influences on the life and work of Hughlings Jackson, Samuel Greenblatt gives an account of Hughlings Jackson's signed works from 1861 to 1864.[138] Greenblatt excludes unsigned papers, some of which were subsequently acknowledged by Hughlings Jackson and therefore can reliably be attributed to him.

We have compiled a complete catalogue raisonné of Hughlings Jackson's writings. We began by collecting all the articles mentioned in Broadbent, Taylor and Greenblatt. Comparing the articles to their entries in the published bibliographies, we found Greenblatt's bibliography to be accurate, though we were able to add several items. On the other hand, we found many inaccuracies in Broadbent and Taylor. Titles of some articles were incorrect, journal references were inaccurate, and some entries could not be found at the place cited. Additionally, careful comparison of papers cited as being published identically in several journals showed them to be, in fact, not identical.

We then examined the original periodicals in which these articles appeared, and collected other works not mentioned by the previous bibliographers. In examining our collection, we found internal references to a number of articles of which Hughlings Jackson claimed authorship, but which have no by-line. Having collected these items, we classified each article by date of publication and source periodical. We assigned each item a unique identification number, comprising the year of publication followed by the number of the item in that year in order of date of publication. If a paper was read on a certain date but published later, we used the date of publication as the assigned date. We treated each part of multiple-published lectures and papers as an individual article.

We found that some items tabulated as being Hughlings Jackson's personal writing are actually reports by unnamed third parties. These were often reports of lectures, or of Hughlings Jackson's comments at medical meetings. Therefore, we classified each paper by the type of by-line. We then assorted them into exclusive categories of by-lined articles, case reports, letters, chapters in multi-authored textbooks, pamphlets, case reports under his care, unsigned editorials which he later claimed, and third person commentaries.

We found 537 articles by and about Hughlings Jackson published between 1861 and 1911. As might be expected, he published the majority of these papers between the ages of thirty and forty-five (1866–1880). He produced 352 by-lined articles, 78 cases under his care, 14 by-lined letters and 2 by-lined chapters in multi-authored texts. He wrote 4 unsigned editorials for which he later claimed authorship. Seventy-nine articles reported his lectures and opinions. We found 8 unsigned articles that he claimed elsewhere.

Virtually all the papers that we collected were written by Hughlings Jackson alone, but we found 18 which he wrote with a collaborator. Early in his career he wrote two papers with J Lockhart Clarke, in both of which Hughlings Jackson was the second author. He also published a case report in which Lockhart Clarke reported the pathological findings. Later

---

[137] Hughlings Jackson, op. cit., note 131 above.
[138] Greenblatt, op. cit., note 3 above, pp. 374–376.

Table 3
Citations by source periodical

Periodicals	Citations
Medical Times and Gazette	136
Lancet	117
British Medical Journal	104
Medical Press and Circular	53
Brain	33
Reports, Royal London Ophthalmic Hospital	14
Medical Examiner	11
London Medical Record	10
Transactions, Ophthalmological Society of the United Kingdom	8
Clinical Lectures and Reports. London Hospital	7
Journal of Mental Science	7
Proceedings, Medical Society of London	7
West Riding Lunatic Asylum Medical Reports	5
Transactions, St Andrews Medical Graduates' Association	3
Transactions of the International Medical Congress. Seventh Session, 1881	3
Medical Mirror	2
The Polyclinic	2
Reynolds System of Medicine	2
Transactions, Clinical Society of London	2
Edinburgh Medical Journal	1
Illustrated Medical News	1
Journal of Psychological Medicine and Mental Pathology	1
London Hospital Gazette	1

Table 3 continued

Periodicals	Citations
Medical Record (NY)	1
Medico-Chirurgical Transactions. Royal Medical and Chirurgical Society of London	1
Ophthalmic Review	1
The Popular Science Monthly	1
La Revue Scientifique de la France et de l'Etranger	1
Transactions, Medical Society of London	1
Transactions of the Obstetrical Society	1
Total	537

in his career he wrote three papers with his student and biographer James Taylor, once as the second author. He was the first author in papers with C E Beevor, J Galloway, J S Risien Russell, W S Colman, P Stewart, J S Collier, H D Singer, S Barnes and J Patton. Cases under his care were reported by R Atkinson and W H R Rivers. One case under the joint care of Hughlings Jackson and Morell Mackenzie was reported. Hughlings Jackson was first author of a 1900 letter to the editor of the *Lancet*, protesting the governance of the National Hospital for the Paralysed and Epileptic, which was signed by seventeen other physicians and surgeons including Gowers, Ferrier, Horsley and Marcus Gunn.[139]

Table 3 shows the distribution of Hughlings Jackson's writings according to the original source periodical.

Sixty-five per cent of Hughlings Jackson's output was published in the *Medical Times and Gazette*, the *Lancet* or the *British Medical Journal*; 81 per cent in these three and *Medical Press and Circular* and *Brain*. Two were published in New York journals, *Popular Science Monthly* and the *Medical Record*; one was published, in French, in *La Revue Scientifique de la France et de l'Etranger*.

Hughlings Jackson and Jonathan Hutchinson edited a by-lined column in the weekly *Medical Times and Gazette* entitled 'Reports of hospital practice in medicine and surgery', from 19 January 1861 to 3 January 1863. This column contained reports of cases, under the care of various physicians, in London and provincial hospitals. Eleven of these case reports carry the initials JHJ, confirming Hughlings Jackson's authorship. Taylor names an additional nine case reports, two of which also appear in Broadbent, which carry no authorial identification other than appearing in a column under Hutchinson and Hughlings Jackson's joint by-line. Both Taylor and Broadbent knew Hughlings Jackson personally and would have had the opportunity to ask him whether he had written these disputed works. Unhappily, there is no record of such an event, and authorship of the disputed case reports remains

---

[139] J Hughlings Jackson, T Buzzard, R Brudenell Carter, *et al.*, 'The medical staff and the management of the National Hospital for the Paralysed and Epileptic, Queen Square', *Lancet*, 1900, **ii**: 351–352.

Introduction

unclear. We have therefore excluded these case reports from our catalogue because their authorship is uncertain.

We have identified 84 pieces not previously attributed to Hughlings Jackson by other bibliographers. These include by-lined letters, original articles and third person commentaries. Many of them describe his comments as president of the Ophthalmological Society of the United Kingdom and the Medical Society of London. They may be a rich source of information about how his works were received by wider medical audiences.

This catalogue raisonné of Hughlings Jackson's published writings includes virtually all his autograph work, excluding only a handful of letters to relatives which are in private hands. It also includes most of the writings about him and his ideas which appeared in British medical periodicals during his lifetime. Our bibliography also illuminates an aspect of Hughlings Jackson's personality which runs contrary to the portrait presented by his biographers. He is often portrayed as lonely, withdrawn, anti-social and modest beyond reason. However, at the zenith of his career he was a familiar figure at medical meetings in London and contributed to many of them. He was elected president of at least four medical societies. When the medical staff of the National Hospital made a public complaint about the governance of the hospital, he was the first signatory of the published letter of protest. He was willing to speak his mind, forcefully if necessary. His lifelong friend, Jonathan Hutchinson, reminds us that he was very much aware of his own intellectual gifts.

What emerges is a picture of a committed physician with few cultural interests but who enjoyed the company of other physicians. He was polite, humble and thoughtful, but was not given to expressions of false modesty. He would not have denied his own talents, such as intelligence or creativity. He was both professionally and intellectually ambitious, a trait which he never denied. Like many productive scientists, he was essentially benevolent in his later years, but we should not overlook his powerful commitment or determination to succeed both personally and professionally.

Catalogue Raisonné of the Writings of John Hughlings Jackson

Key

Unique identification number Taylor citation (T) Broadbent citation (B) Greenblatt citation (G) Location in *Selected Writings* (SW)	Title Authorial identifier	Periodical source Date of publication

(T) J Hughlings Jackson, *Neurological fragments*, with 'Biographical Memoir' and 'List of Dr Hughlings Jackson's Published Writings', by James Taylor, London, Humphrey Milford and Oxford University Press, 1925, pp. 205–221.

(B) William Broadbent, 'Hughlings Jackson as a pioneer in nervous physiology and pathology', *Brain*, 1903, **26**: 305–366, pp. 356–366

(G) Samuel H Greenblatt, 'The major influences on the early life and work of John Hughlings Jackson', *Bull Hist Med*, 1965, **39**: 374–376.

(SW) *Selected writings of John Hughlings Jackson*, edited by James Taylor, with the advice and assistance of Gordon Holmes and F M R Walshe, 2 vols, London, Hodder and Stoughton, 1931–1932.

Writings of John Hughlings Jackson

1861

ID	TITLE	PERIODICAL SOURCE
61–01 T61 B1	Cases of abscess in the brain Unsigned, but claimed in first person plural in *Med Times Gaz*, 1862, **ii**: 221–226, on p. 221.	*Med Times Gaz*, 1861, **i**: 196–200 23 Feb 61
61–02 T61 G1 B2	Syphilitic affections of the nervous system. Cases of epilepsy associated with syphilis Initialled report.	*Med Times Gaz*, 1861, **i**: 648–652 22 June 61
61–03 T61 G1 B2	Syphilitic affections of the nervous system. Cases of epilepsy associated with syphilis Initialled report.	*Med Times Gaz*, 1861, **ii**: 59–60 20 July 61
61–04 T61 G1	Syphilitic affections of the nervous system. Cases of paralysis associated with syphilis Unsigned report; *Med Times Gaz*, 1861, **ii**: 133–135, which is initialled, is marked as "continuation from p. 85".	*Med Times Gaz*, 1861, **ii**: 83–85 7 July 61
61–05 T61 G1	Syphilitic affections of the nervous system. Cases of paralysis associated with syphilis Initialled report.	*Med Times Gaz*, 1861, **ii**: 133–135 10 Aug 61
61–06 T61 G4	Cases of reflex (?) amaurosis with coloured vision By-line.	*Royal London Ophthalmic Hospital Reports*, 1861, **3**: 286–291 Issue dated Oct 61
61–07 G1	Syphilitic affections of the nervous system. Cases of paralysis associated with syphilis Initialled report.	*Med Times Gaz*, 1861, **ii**: 456 2 Nov 61

ID	TITLE	PERIODICAL SOURCE
61–08 T61 G1	Syphilitic affections of the nervous system. Cases of amaurosis in connexion with syphilis Initialled report.	*Med Times Gaz*, 1861, **ii**: 502–503 16 Nov 61
61–09 T61 G2	Cases of deafness associated with syphilis Initialled report.	*Med Times Gaz*, 1861, **ii**: 530–531 23 Nov 61
61–10 T61 G3	Cases of paralysis of the portio dura Initialled report.	*Med Times Gaz*, 1861, **ii**: 606–608 14 Dec 61

1862

ID	TITLE	PERIODICAL SOURCE
62–01	Apoplexy of the pons Varolii—Recovery—"Fit" (Nineteen years ago) followed by paralysis of the external recti and of the Face and Trunk both motion and sensation—Gradual recovery—Clinical remarks (case under the care of Dr. Brown-Séquard) Unsigned, claimed in *Clinical Lectures and Reports by the Medical and Surgical Staff of the London Hospital* 1864, **1**: 346, with same title, journal and year but incorrect month (given as Feb, actually Apr).	*Med Times Gaz*, 1862, **i**: 429–430 26 Apr 62
62–02 G5	Cases of disease of the cerebellum Initialled report.	*Med Times Gaz*, 1862, **ii**: 221–226 30 Aug 62
62–03 G5	Cases of disease of the cerebellum Initialled report.	*Med Times Gaz*, 1862, **ii**: 407–409 10 Oct 62
62–04 G6	Cases of injury of the spine and of diseases of the spinal cord Initialled report.	*Med Times Gaz*, 1862, **ii**: 463–465 1 Nov 62
62–05 G8	Metropolitan Free Hospital. Sequelae of scarlet fever (Under the care of Dr. Hughlings Jackson) Case under the care of HJ.	*Med Times Gaz*, 1862, **ii**: 575 29 Nov 62
62–06 G7	The ophthalmoscope, as an aid to the study of diseases of the brain By-line.	*Med Times Gaz*, 1862, **ii**: 598–601 12 Dec 62

1863

ID	TITLE	PERIODICAL SOURCE
63–01 G9	Cases of injury of the spine and of diseases of the spinal cord Unsigned, but labelled as continuation from *Med Times Gaz*, 1862, **ii**: 463–465.	*Med Times Gaz*, 1863, **i**: 31–33 10 Jan 63
63–02 G11	Hospital for the Epileptic and Paralysed. Convulsive spasms of the right hand and arm preceding epileptic seizures (Case under the care of Dr. Hughlings Jackson) Case under the care of HJ.	*Med Times Gaz*, 1863, **i**: 110–111 31 Jan 63
63–03 T63 G12 B4	Metropolitan Free Hospital. Syphilis, followed by unilateral convulsions four months afterwards—temporary hemiplegia—paralysis of the sixth nerve on the same side—recovery (Under the care of Dr. Hughlings Jackson) Case under the care of HJ.	*Med Times Gaz*, 1863, **i**: 111 31 Jan 63
63–04	Cases of disease of the pons Varolii Unsigned, claimed first person singular in *Clinical Lectures and Reports by the Medical and Surgical Staff of the London Hospital*, 1864, **1**: 337–387, on p. 343.	*Med Times Gaz*, 1863, **i**: 210–215 28 Feb 63
63–05	Hospital for the Epileptic and Paralysed. Severe pain at the back of the head, and frequent vomiting, followed in a few months by complete amaurosis—epileptiform convulsions and partial paralysis (Under the care of Dr. Brown-Séquard; communicated by Dr. Hughlings Jackson, Assistant-Physician at the Hospital) Case under the care of Brown-Séquard, communicated by HJ.	*Med Times Gaz*, 1863, **i**: 533. 23 May 63

ID	TITLE	PERIODICAL SOURCE
63–06	Hospital for the Epileptic and Paralysed. Vomiting and headache followed by amaurosis and epileptiform seizures—increase in size of the head (Under the care of Dr. Hughlings Jackson)	*Med Times Gaz*, 1863, **i**: 533.
	Case under the care of HJ.	23 May 63
63–07 T63 G13 B5 SW1, p. 1	Hospital for the Epileptic and Paralysed. Unilateral epileptiform seizures, attended by temporary defect of sight (Under the care of Dr. Hughlings Jackson)	*Med Times Gaz*, 1863, **i**: 588.
	Case under the care of HJ.	6 June 63
63–08 T63 G14 B6 SW1, pp. 1–2	Metropolitan Free Hospital. Epileptiform seizures—aura from the thumb—attacks of coloured vision (Under the care of Dr. Hughlings Jackson)	*Med Times Gaz*, 1863, **i**: 589
	Case under the care of HJ.	6 June 63
63–09 G15	Hospital for the Epileptic and Paralysed. Hemiplegia in an old man—recovery—spasm of the face (Under the care of Dr. Hughlings Jackson)	*Med Times Gaz*, 1863, **ii**: 11–12
	Case under the care of HJ.	4 July 63
63–10 G16	Hospital for the Epileptic and Paralysed. Epilepsy following some months after injury to the head (Under the care of Dr. Hughlings Jackson)	*Med Times Gaz*, 1863, **ii**: 65
	Case under the care of HJ.	18 July 63
63–11 T63 G17 B7	Hospital for the Epileptic and Paralysed. Epileptiform convulsions (unilateral) after an injury to the head (Under the care of Dr. Hughlings Jackson)	*Med Times Gaz*, 1863, **ii**: 65–66
	Case under the care of HJ.	18 July 63

ID	TITLE	PERIODICAL SOURCE
63–12 T63 G18	An experimental inquiry into the effect of the application of ice to the back of the neck on the retinal circulation By-line.	*Med Times Gaz*, 1863, **ii**: 90–91 25 July 63
63–13 T63 G19	Hospital for the Epileptic and Paralysed. Notes on the use of the ophthalmoscope in affections of the nervous system (Communicated by Dr. Hughlings Jackson, Assistant-Physician to the Hospital) Communicated by HJ.	*Med Times Gaz*, 1863, **ii**: 359 3 Oct 63
63–14 T63 B8	Unilateral chorea, interstitial keratitis; slow recovery under the use of iodide of potassium (Under the care of Dr. Hughlings Jackson) Case under the care of HJ.	*Med Times Gaz*, 1863, **ii**: 407–408 17 Oct 63
63–15 T63 G20 B9	The London Hospital. Giddiness, pain in the head, and vomiting coming on suddenly—amaurosis—no paralysis—death eleven weeks after the first seizure—autopsy—apoplexy in middle cerebral lobe (Under the care of Dr. Hughlings Jackson) Case under the care of HJ.	*Med Times Gaz*, 1863, **ii**: 588–589 5 Dec 63
63–16 T63 G21 B10	Observations on defects of sight in brain disease By-line.	*Royal London Ophthalmic Hospital Reports*, 1863, **4**: 10–19 Edition printed 1863
63–17 T63 G22	Ophthalmoscopic examination during sleep By-line.	*Royal London Ophthalmic Hospital Reports*, 1863, **4**: 35–37 Edition printed 1863

1864

ID	TITLE	PERIODICAL SOURCE
64–01 T64 G23 B14	Hospital for Epilepsy and Paralysis. Clinical remarks on hemiplegia, with loss of speech—its association with valvular disease of the heart (Cases under the care of Dr. Hughlings Jackson) Cases under the care of HJ.	*Med Times Gaz*, 1864, **i**: 123 30 Jan 64
64–02 T64 G24 B15	Hospital for Epilepsy and Paralysis. Clinical remarks on defects of sight in diseases of the nervous system (Cases under the care of Dr. Hughlings Jackson) Cases under the care of HJ.	*Med Times Gaz*, 1864, **i**: 480–482 30 Apr 64
64–03 T64 G25 B16	Hemiplegia on the right side, with loss of speech By-lined letter.	*Br Med J*, 1864, **i**: 572–573 21 May 64
64–04 T64 G26	Note on amaurosis in hemiplegia By-line.	*Med Times Gaz*, 1864, **ii**: 87 23 July 64
64–05 T64 G27 B17 SW1, pp. 3–4	The London Hospital. Loss of speech, with hemiplegia on the left side—valvular disease—epileptiform seizures affecting the side paralysed (Under the care of Dr. Hughlings Jackson) Case under the care of HJ.	*Med Times Gaz*, 1864, **ii**: 166–167 13 Aug 64
64–06 T64 G28 B18	Hospital for Epilepsy and Paralysis. Epileptic aphemia with epileptic seizures on the right side (Under the care of Dr. Hughlings Jackson) Case under the care of HJ.	*Med Times Gaz*, 1864, **ii**: 167–168 13 Aug 64

ID	TITLE	PERIODICAL SOURCE
64–07 T64 G29	Unilateral epileptiform seizures beginning by a disagreeable smell Case under the care of HJ.	*Med Times Gaz*, 1864, **ii**: 168 13 Aug 64
64–08 T64 G32 B11	On the study of diseases of the nervous system. A lecture delivered June, 1864 By-line.	*Clinical Lectures and Reports by the Medical and Surgical Staff of the London Hospital*, 1864, **1**: 146–158 Must be after June 64 and before review published 5 Nov 64 (64–11). Volume printed 1864
64–09 T64 G33 B12	Illustrations of diseases of the nervous system By-line.	*Clinical Lectures and Reports by the Medical and Surgical Staff of the London Hospital*, 1864, **1**: 337–387 Must be before review published 5 Nov 64 (64–11). Volume printed 1864

ID	TITLE	PERIODICAL SOURCE
64–10 T64 G34 B13	Loss of speech: its association with valvular disease of the heart, and with hemiplegia on the right side—Defects of smell—Defects of speech in chorea—Arterial regions in epilepsy By-line.	*Clinical Lectures and Reports by the Medical and Surgical Staff of the London Hospital*, 1864, **1**: 388–471 Must be before review published 5 Nov 64 (64–11). Volume printed 1864
64–11	Reviews and Notices. Clinical Lectures and Reports by the Medical and Surgical Staff of the London Hospital Report of Hughlings Jackson's views.	*Br Med J*, 1864, **ii**: 524 5 Nov 64
64–12 T64 G30 B19	National Hospital for Epilepsy and Paralysis. Clinical remarks on cases of defects of expression (by words, writing, signs, etc.) in diseases of the nervous system (Under the care of Dr. Hughlings Jackson) Cases under the care of HJ.	*Lancet*, 1864, **ii**: 604–605 26 Nov 64
64–13 T64 G31 B20	London Hospital. Chorea, with paralysis, affecting the right side; difficulty in talking (Under the care of Dr. Hughlings Jackson) Cases under the care of HJ.	*Lancet*, 1864, **ii**: 606 26 Nov 64

1865

ID	TITLE	PERIODICAL SOURCE
65–01 T65 B24	The London Hospital. Involuntary ejaculations following fright—subsequently chorea (Under the care of Dr Hughlings Jackson) Case under the care of HJ.	*Med Times Gaz*, 1865, **i**: 89 28 Jan 65
65–02 T65	On a case of disease of the posterior columns of the cord—locomotor ataxy (?) By-line: J Lockhart Clarke and J Hughlings Jackson.	*Lancet*, 1865, **i**: 617–620 10 June 65
65–03 T65 B25	The London Hospital. Tumour at the base of the brain—death—autopsy—clinical remarks. (Under the care of Dr. Hughlings Jackson.) Case under the care of HJ.	*Med Times Gaz*, 1865, **i**: 626–627 17 June 65
65–04 T65 B23	Affections of cranial nerves in locomotor ataxy By-lined letter.	*Lancet*, 1865, **ii**: 247–248 26 Aug 65
65–05 T65 B22	Hospital for the Epileptic and Paralysed. Hemiplegia on the right side, with deficit of speech—death—autopsy. (Under the care of Dr Hughlings Jackson) Case under the care of HJ.	*Med Times Gaz*, 1865, **ii**: 283–284 9 Sept 65
65–06 T65 B21	Lectures on hemiplegia By-line.	*Clinical Lectures and Reports by the Medical and Surgical Staff of the London Hospital*, 1865, **2**: 297–332 Volume printed 1865

ID	TITLE	PERIODICAL SOURCE
65–07 T63 B26	Observations on defects of sight in diseases of the nervous system By-line.	*Royal London Ophthalmic Hospital Reports,* 1865, **4**: 389–446 Edition dated 1865
65–08 T63 B26	Observations on defects of sight in diseases of the nervous system By-line	*Royal London Ophthalmic Hospital Reports,* 1865, **5**: 51–78 Edition dated 1865

1866

ID	TITLE	PERIODICAL SOURCE
66–01 T66	The London Hospital. Clinical remarks on emotional and intellectual language in some cases of disease of the nervous system (Under the care of Dr. Hughlings Jackson) Case under the care of HJ.	*Lancet*, 1866, **i**: 174–176 17 Feb 66
66–02 T66 B29	Note on lateral deviation of the eyes in hemiplegia and in certain epileptiform seizures By-line.	*Lancet*, 1866, **i**: 311–312 24 Mar 66
66–03 T66 B30	London Hospital. A case of progressive locomotor ataxy: loss of smell and hearing; defect of sight, with atrophy of the optic discs; variocele and atrophy of the testes (Under the care of Dr. Hughlings Jackson) Case under the care of HJ.	*Lancet*, 1866, **i**: 345–346 31 Mar 66
66–04 T66 B31	National Hospital for the Epileptic and Paralysed. Clinical remarks on cases of temporary loss of speech and power of expression (epileptic aphemia? Aphrasia? Aphasia?) and on epilepsies (Under the care of Dr. Hughlings Jackson) Case under the care of HJ.	*Med Times Gaz*, 1866, **i**: 442–443 28 Apr 66
66–05 T66	National Hospital for the Epileptic and Paralysed. Clinical remarks on the occasional occurrence of subjective sensations of smell in patients who are liable to epileptiform seizures, or who have symptoms of mental derangement, and in others (Under the care of Dr. Hughlings Jackson) Case under the care of HJ	*Lancet*, 1866, **i**: 659–660 16 June 66
66–06 T66 B32 SW2, pp. 121–128	Notes on the physiology and pathology of language. Remarks on those cases of disease of the nervous system in which defect of expression is the most striking symptom By-line.	*Med Times Gaz*, 1866, **i**: 659–662 23 June 66

ID	TITLE	PERIODICAL SOURCE
66–07 T66 B33	On a case of loss of power of expression; inability to talk, to write, and to read correctly after convulsive attacks By-line.	*Br Med J*, 1866, **ii**: 92–94 28 July 66
66–08 T66	Hemiplegia of the left side, with defect of speech By-lined letter.	*Med Times Gaz*, 1866, **ii**: 210 25 Aug 66
66–09 T66 B34	Tobacco smoking in diseases of the nervous system. Sex in diseases of the nervous system. The form of amaurosis complicating locomotor ataxy By-line.	*Med Times Gaz*, 1866, **ii**: 219–222 1 Sept 66
66–10 T66 B33	On a case of loss of power of expression; inability to talk, to write, and to read correctly after convulsive attacks By-line.	*Br Med J*, 1866, **ii**: 326–330 22 Sept 66
66–11 T66 B35	London Hospital. Case of disease of cerebral arteries (syphilitic?); softening of the brain; clinical remarks (Under the care of Dr. Hughlings Jackson) Cases under the care of HJ.	*Lancet*, 1866, **ii**: 467–468 27 Oct 66
66–12	Reports of Societies. Harveian Society of London. Oct. 18th, 1866 Report of Hughlings Jackson's comments on a paper on the causes of insanity, by Henry Maudsley.	*Br Med J*, 1866, **ii**: 586–590, on p. 587 24 Nov 66
66–13	The National Hospital for the Epileptic and Paralyzed. The electrical room Unsigned, claimed in first person singular at *Royal London Ophthalmic Hospital Reports*, 1866, **5**: 251–306, on p. 267.	*Med Times Gaz*, 1866, **ii**: 583–585 1 Dec 66

ID	TITLE	PERIODICAL SOURCE
66–14 T66 B36	London Hospital. Case of disease of the left side of the brain, involving corpus striatum, etc.; the aphasia of Trousseau; clinical remarks on psychico-physical symptoms (Under the care of Dr. Hughlings Jackson) Case under the care of HJ.	*Lancet*, 1866, **ii**: 605–606 1 Dec 66
66–15 T66 B26	A physician's notes on ophthalmoscopy—cases of disease of the nervous system in which there were defects of smell, sight and hearing By-line.	*Royal London Ophthalmic Hospital Reports*, 1866, **5**: 251–306 Volume printed 1866
66–16 T66 B27	A lecture on cases of cerebral haemorrhage By-line.	*Clinical Lectures and Reports by the Medical and Surgical Staff of the London Hospital*, 1866, **3**: 237–258 Volume printed 1866
66–17 T66 B28	Note on the functions of the optic thalamus By-line.	*Clinical Lectures and Reports by the Medical and Surgical Staff of the London Hospital*, 1866, **3**: 373–377 Volume printed 1866
66–18	Amaurosis. Tumour at the base of the brain—death—autopsy—clinical remarks By-line.	*Ophthalmic Rev*, 1866, **2**: 288–290 Volume printed 1866

1867

ID	TITLE	PERIODICAL SOURCE
67–01 T67 B37 SW1, pp. 5–6	Note on the comparison and contrast of regional palsy and spasm By-line.	*Lancet*, 1867, **i**: 205 16 Feb 67
67–02 T67 B37 SW1, pp. 5–6	Note on the comparison and contrast of regional palsy and spasm By-line.	*Lancet*, 1867, **i**: 295–297 9 Mar 67
67–03 T67 B38	London Hospital. Choreal movements of the right arm and leg in a man seventy-four years of age: clinical remarks on cases of chorea (Under the care of Dr. Hughlings Jackson) Case under the care of HJ.	*Br Med J*, 1867, **i**: 570–572 18 May 67
67–04 T67	The ophthalmoscope in physicians' practice By-lined letter.	*Br Med J*, 1867, **i**: 722 15 June 67
67–05	National Hospital for the Epileptic and Paralysed. Notes on cases of diseases of the nervous system (Under the care of Dr. Hughlings Jackson) Case under the care of HJ	*Br Med J*, 1867, **ii**: 472–474 23 Nov 67
67–06	National Hospital for the Epileptic and Paralysed. Notes on cases of diseases of the nervous system (Under the care of Dr. Hughlings Jackson) Case under the care of HJ.	*Br Med J*, 1867, **ii**: 499–500 30 Nov 67
67–07 T67 B39	Remarks on the disorderly movements of chorea and convulsion By-line.	*Med Times Gaz*, 1867, **ii**: 642–643 24 Dec 67

ID	TITLE	PERIODICAL SOURCE
67–08 T67 B39	Remarks on the disorderly movements of chorea and convulsion, and on localisation By-line.	*Med Times Gaz*, 1867, **ii**: 669–670 21 Dec 67
67–09 T67	Note on regional palsy and spasm By-line.	*Br Med J*, 1867, **ii**: 587 28 Dec 67
67–10	Notes of hospital cases Cases under the care of HJ, reported by Mr. Frederick Mackenzie.	*Royal London Ophthalmic Hospital Reports*, 1867, **6**: 50–53 Volume printed 1867
67–11 T67 B40	Cases of disease of the nervous system By-line.	*Clinical Lectures and Reports by the Medical and Surgical Staff of the London Hospital*, 1867, **4**: 314–394 Volume dated 1867–68
67–12	On a case of muscular atrophy, with disease of the spinal cord and medulla oblongata. By-line: J Lockhart Clarke and J Hughlings Jackson.	*Trans Medico-Chirurgical Society of London*, series 2, 1867, **32**: 489–499 Received 28 May 67. Read 25 June 67

1868

ID	TITLE	PERIODICAL SOURCE
68–01 T68 B41	On latency of optic neuritis in cerebral disease By-line.	*Med Times Gaz*, 1868, **i**: 143 8 Feb 68
68–02	London Hospital. Case of occasional loss of consciousness, with subjective sensations of smell (Under the care of Dr. Hughlings Jackson) Case under the care of HJ.	*Med Times Gaz*, 1868, **i**: 231 29 Feb 68
68–03 T68 B42	London Hospital. Aphasia with hemiplegia of the left side (Under the care of Dr. Hughlings Jackson) Case under the care of HJ.	*Lancet*, 1868, **i**: 316 7 May 68
68–04	Hospital for the Epileptic and Paralysed. The ophthalmoscope in physicians' practice: Clinical remarks on cases of optic neuritis in brain-disease (Under the care of Dr. Hughlings Jackson) Case under the care of HJ.	*Br Med J*, 1868, **i**: 300 28 Mar 68
68–05 T68	Defect of intellectual expression (aphasia) with left hemiplegia By-lined letter.	*Lancet*, 1868, **i**: 457 4 Apr 68
68–06 T68	The London Hospital. Case of severe brain disease with double optic neuritis (Under the care of Dr. Hughlings Jackson) Case under the care of HJ.	*Med Times Gaz*, 1868, **i**: 392 17 Apr 68
68–07 T68 B44	National Hospital for the Epileptic and Paralysed. Case of convulsive attacks arrested by stopping the aura (Under the care of Dr. Hughlings Jackson) Case under the care of HJ.	*Lancet*, 1868, **i**: 618–619 16 May 68

ID	TITLE	PERIODICAL SOURCE
68–08 T68 B43	The London Hospital. Clinical remarks on cases of convulsions beginning unilaterally with double optic neuritis (Under the care of Dr. Hughlings Jackson) Case under the care of HJ.	*Med Times Gaz*, 1868, **i:** 524–525 16 May 68
68–09	Syphilitic affections of the nervous system Unsigned but claimed in first person singular in *Lancet*, 1880, **i:** 357–359, on p. 358.	*Med Times Gaz*, 1868, **i:** 551–553 23 May 68
68–10 T68	The ophthalmoscope in pyaemia By-lined letter.	*Med Times Gaz*, 1868, **i:** 653 13 June 68
68–11	Reports of Societies. Obstetrical Society of London. Wednesday July 1, 1868. Chorea in pregnancy Report of Hughlings Jackson's comments on a paper on chorea in pregnancy by Dr Barnes.	*Med Times Gaz*, 1868, **ii:** 137–138 1 Aug 68
68–12 T68 B45 SW2, pp. 215–237	Notes on the physiology and pathology of the nervous system By-line.	*Med Times Gaz*, 1868, **ii:** 177–179 15 Aug 68
68–13 T68 B45 SW2, pp. 215–237	Notes on the physiology and pathology of the nervous system By-line.	*Med Times Gaz*, 1868, **ii:** 208–209 22 Aug 68
68–14 T68	Dr. Hughlings Jackson, F.R.C.P., on the physiology of language Report of Hughlings Jackson's talk at the British Association for the Advancement of Science at Norwich, August 1868.	*Med Times Gaz*, 1868, **ii:** 275–276 5 Sep 68

ID	TITLE	PERIODICAL SOURCE
68–15 T68	Reports of Societies. British Association for the Advancement of Science. Section II—Biology: Department of anatomy and physiology. The physiology of language Report of Hughlings Jackson's talk at the British Association for the Advancement of Science at Norwich, August 1868.	*Br Med J*, 1868, **ii**: 259 5 Sep 68
68–16 T68	The physiology of language By-line.	*Med Press Circular*, 1868, **6**: 237–239 9 Sep 68
68–17 T68 B45 SW2, pp. 215–237	Notes on the physiology and pathology of the nervous system By-line.	*Med Times Gaz*, 1868, **ii**: 358–359 26 Sep 68
68–18 T68 B45 SW2, pp. 238–245	Observations on the physiology and pathology of hemi-chorea By-line.	*Edinburgh Med J*, 1868, **14**: 294–303 issue dated Oct 68
68–19 T68	Chorea in pregnancy By-lined letter.	*Med Times Gaz*, 1868, **ii**: 410 3 Oct 68
68–20	National Hospital for the Epileptic and Paralysed. Syphilitic disease of the brain; optic neuritis; convulsions beginning unilaterally (Under the care of Dr. Hughlings Jackson) Case under the care of HJ.	*Lancet*, 1868, **ii**: 539–540 24 Oct 68
68–21 T68 B45 SW2, pp. 215–237	Notes on the physiology and pathology of the nervous system By-line.	*Med Times Gaz*, 1868, **ii**: 526–528 7 Nov 68

ID	TITLE	PERIODICAL SOURCE
68–22 T68 B45 SW2, pp. 215–237	Notes on the physiology and pathology of the nervous system By-line.	*Med Times Gaz*, 1868, **ii**: 696 19 Dec 68
68–23 T68	Cases of disease of the nervous system in patients the subjects of inherited syphilis By-line.	*St Andrews Medical Graduates' Association Transactions, 1867*, 146–160. Volume printed 1868
68–24	A case of epileptiform amaurosis By-line.	*Royal London Ophthalmic Hospital Reports*, 1868, **6**: 131–135 Volume printed 1868
68–25 T68 B48	Convulsions By-lined chapter in multi-author textbook.	*A system of medicine*, J R Reynolds (ed.), 1868, **2**: 217–250. Volume printed 1868
68–26 T68 B47	On apoplexy and cerebral hemorrhage By-lined chapter in multi-author textbook.	*A system of medicine*, J R Reynolds (ed.), 1868, **2**: 504–543 Volume printed 1868

1869

ID	TITLE	PERIODICAL SOURCE
69–01 T69 B50 SW2, pp. 246–250	Abstract of the Gulstonian [sic] lectures on certain points in the study and classification of diseases of the nervous system. Delivered at the Royal College of Physicians By-line.	*Lancet*, 1869, **i**: 307–308 27 Feb 69
69–02 T69 B50 SW2, pp. 246–250	Gulstonian [sic] lectures on certain points in the study and classification of diseases of the nervous system. Delivered at the Royal College of Physicians By-line.	*Br Med J*, 1869, **i**: 184 27 Feb 69
69–03 T69 B50 SW2, pp. 246–250	Abstract of the Gulstonian lectures on certain points in the study and classification of diseases of the nervous system. Delivered at the Royal College of Physicians By-line.	*Lancet*, 1869, **i**: 344–345 6 Mar 69
69–04 T69 B50 SW2, pp. 246–250	Gulstonian lectures on certain points in the study and classification of diseases of the nervous system. Delivered at the Royal College of Physicians By-line.	*Br Med J*, 1869, **i**: 210 6 Mar 69
69–05 T69 B51 SW2, pp. 215–237	Notes on the physiology and pathology of the nervous system By-line.	*Med Times Gaz*, 1869, **i**: 245–246 6 Mar 69
69–06 T69 B50 SW2, pp. 246–250	Abstract of the Gulstonian lectures on certain points in the study and classification of diseases of the nervous system. Delivered at the Royal College of Physicians By-line.	*Lancet*, 1869, **i**: 379–380 13 Mar 69
69–07 T69 B50 SW2, pp. 246–250	Gulstonian lectures on certain points in the study and classification of diseases of the nervous system. Delivered at the Royal College of Physicians By-line.	*Br Med J*, 1869, **i**: 236 13 Mar 69

ID	TITLE	PERIODICAL SOURCE
69–08	Cases of disease of the nervous system in patients the subjects of inherited syphilis Review of pamphlet written by HJ.	*Lancet*, 1869, **i**: 498 10 Apr 69
69–09 T69 B53 SW2, pp. 215–237	Notes on the physiology and pathology of the nervous system By-line.	*Med Times Gaz*, 1869, **i**: 600 5 June 69
69–10 T69 B52	Hospital for the Epileptic and Paralysed. Epileptic or epileptiform seizures occurring with discharge from the ear (Cases under the care of Dr. Hughlings Jackson) Case under the care of HJ.	*Br Med J*, 1869, **i**: 591 26 June 69
69–11 T69 B49	Report of a case of disease of one lobe of the cerebrum, and of both lobes of the cerebellum By-line.	*Med Mirror*, 1869, **6**: 126–127 1 Sept 69
69–12 B49	The function of the cerebellum By-line.	*Med Mirror*, 1869, **6**: 138–140 and 147 1 Oct 69
69–13 T69 B55 SW2, pp. 215–237	Notes on the physiology and pathology of the nervous system By-line.	*Med Times Gaz*, 1869, **ii**: 481–482 23 Oct 69
69–14 T69 B56	London Hospital. Death by haemorrhage from cerebral tumours (Under the care of Dr. Hughlings Jackson) Case under the care of HJ.	*Lancet*, 1869, **ii**: 571–572 23 Oct 69
69–15 T69 B58	London Hospital. Lateral deviation of the eyes in cases of hemiplegia By-line.	*Lancet*, 1869, **ii**: 672 13 Nov 69

ID	TITLE	PERIODICAL SOURCE
69–16 T69 B57	National Hospital for the Epileptic and Paralysed. Remarks on an association of nervous symptoms which frequently depends on intracranial syphilitic disease By-line.	*Lancet*, 1869, **ii**: 803 11 Dec 69
69–17	The periscope. Dr. Hughlings Jackson on cerebral disease in connection with ophthalmic symptoms Report of Hughlings Jackson's views, extracted from *Clinical Lectures and Reports by the Medical and Surgical Staff of the London Hospital*, 1867, **4**: 314–394.	*Royal London Ophthalmic Hospital Reports*, 1869, **6**: 240 Issue dated 1869
69–18	On chorea in pregnancy By Robert Barnes, who discusses Hughlings Jackson's views.	*Trans Obstet Soc London*, 1869, **10**: 147–195 Volume printed 1869

1870

ID	TITLE	PERIODICAL SOURCE
70–01 T70 B59	The London Hospital. Case of palsies of several cranial nerves, including the nerves to the larynx, all on the left side—weakness of the limbs of the right side (Under the care of Dr. Hughlings Jackson and Dr. Morell Mackenzie) Cases under the care of HJ and Dr Morell Mackenzie.	*Med Times Gaz*, 1870, **i**: 34–35 8 Jan 70
70–02 T70	Reports of Societies. Clinical Society Report of case presentation by HJ on optic neuritis and focal seizures	*Med Times Gaz*, 1870, **i**: 480–481 30 Apr 70
70–03	Remarks on tongue-biting in convulsions By-line.	*Br Med J*, 1870, **i**: 409 23 Apr 70
70–04	Reports of Societies. Clinical Society of London Friday April 8th Report of case presentation by HJ.	*Br Med J*, 1870, **i**: 452 30 Apr 70
70–05 T70 B60 B61	Hospital for the Epileptic and Paralysed. Notes on cases of disease of the nervous system (Under the care of Dr. Hughlings Jackson) Cases under the care of HJ.	*Br Med J*, 1870, **ii**: 459–460 29 Oct 70
70–06 T70 SW1, pp. 8–36	A study of convulsions By-line.	*St Andrews Medical Graduates' Association Transactions*, *1869*, **3**: 162–204 Must be before 12 Nov 70. Volume printed 1870

ID	TITLE	PERIODICAL SOURCE
70–07	Reviews and notices of books. A study of convulsions	*Lancet*, 1870, **ii**: 674
	Review of pamphlet reprinted from *St Andrews Medical Graduates' Association Transactions 1869*, 1870, **3**: 162–204.	12 Nov 70

1871

ID	TITLE	PERIODICAL SOURCE
71–01	London Hospital. Notes from the out-patient practice of Dr. Hughlings Jackson Report of HJ's remarks.	*Lancet*, 1871, **i**: 376–377 18 Mar 71
71–02 T71 B63	Case illustrating difficulties in the diagnosis of cerebral haemorrhage and drunkenness By-line.	*Med Times Gaz*, 1871, **i**: 360–361 1 Apr 71
71–03 T71	Defect of hearing in diphtherial paralysis By-lined letter.	*Lancet*, 1871, **i**: 728 27 May 71
71–04 T71 B64	On the routine use of the ophthalmoscope in cases of cerebral disease By-line.	*Med Times Gaz*, 1871, **i**: 627–629 3 June 71
71–05 T71	Reports of Societies. Clinical Society of London Report of HJ's comments on a patient with aphasia and right hemiplegia.	*Med Times Gaz*, 1871, **i**: 702–703 17 June 71
71–06 T71 B65 SW2, pp. 251–264	Lecture on optic neuritis from intracranial disease. Delivered at the London Hospital By-line.	*Med Times Gaz*, 1871, **ii**: 241–243 26 Aug 71
71–07 T71	Tumour of the middle lobe of the cerebellum Report of HJ's paper read at the annual meeting of the British Medical Association, August 1871.	*Br Med J*, 1871, **ii**: 241–243, on p. 242 26 Aug 71

ID	TITLE	PERIODICAL SOURCE
71–08 T71 B65 SW2, pp. 251–264	Lecture on optic neuritis from intracranial disease. Delivered at the London Hospital By-line.	*Med Times Gaz*, 1871, **ii**: 341–342 16 Sept 71
71–09 T71 B66	London Hospital. Case of tumour of the middle lobe of the cerebellum By-line.	*Br Med J*, 1871, **ii**: 528–529 4 Nov 71
71–10 T71 B65 SW2, pp. 251–264	Lecture on optic neuritis from intracranial disease. Delivered at the London Hospital By-line.	*Med Times Gaz*, 1871, **ii**: 581 11 Nov 71
71–11 T71 B67	Hospital for the Epileptic and Paralysed. Notes on cases of disease of the nervous system (Under the care of Dr. Hughlings Jackson) Case under the care of HJ.	*Br Med J*, 1871, **ii**: 641–642 2 Dec 71
71–12 T71 B68	London Hospital. Case of epileptiform seizure, beginning in the right hand (Under the care of Dr. Hughlings-Jackson) Case under the care of HJ.	*Med Times Gaz*, 1871, **ii**: 767–769 23 Dec 71
71–13 B62	Case of hemiplegia in a syphilitic subject. Read May 26, 1870 By-line.	*Trans Clin Soc London,* 1871, **4**: 183–187 Volume printed 1871

1872

ID	TITLE	PERIODICAL SOURCE
72–01 T72	On partial convulsive seizures, with plugging of cerebral veins By-line.	*Med Times Gaz*, 1872, **i**: 4–5 6 Jan 72
72–02 T72	On a case of defect of speech following right-sided convulsion By-line.	*Lancet*, 1872, **i**: 72–73 20 Jan 72
72–03 T72	On partial convulsive seizures, with plugging of cerebral veins By-line.	*Med Times Gaz*, 1872, **i**: 94 27 Jan 72
72–04 T72 B72	London Hospital. Remarks on a case of chorea in a dog By-line.	*Lancet*, 1872, **i**: 148 3 Feb 72
72–05 T72 SW2, pp. 265–269	Abstract of the oration delivered before the Hunterian Society of London, February 7th, 1872. The physiological aspects of education By-line.	*Br Med J*, 1872, **i**: 179–181 17 Feb 72
72–06 T72 SW2, pp. 265–269	Abstract of the Hunterian oration, delivered before the Hunterian Society, Feb 17th, 1872. The physiological aspects of education By-line.	*Lancet*, 1872, **i**: 260 24 Feb 72
72–07 T72	London Hospital. Remarks on difficulties in the diagnosis of the causes of apoplexy By-line.	*Lancet*, 1872, **i**: 505 13 Apr 72
72–08 T72 B69	London Hospital. Case of disease of the brain—left hemiplegia—mental affection (Under the care of Dr. Hughlings-Jackson) Case under the care of HJ.	*Med Times Gaz*, 1872, **i**: 513–514 4 May 72

ID	TITLE	PERIODICAL SOURCE
72–09	National Hospital for Epileptics. Notes of cases under the care of Dr. Hughlings Jackson Case under the care of HJ.	*Br Med J*, 1872, **i**: 526 18 May 72
72–10 T72	London Hospital. Remarks on affections of hearing in cases of disease of the nervous system By-line.	*Med Times Gaz*, 1872, **ii**: 37–39 13 July 72
72–11	Corrigendum By-lined letter.	*Med Times Gaz*, 1872, **ii**: 84 20 July 72
72–12 T72	The London Hospital. Remarks on cases of intracranial tumour (Under the care of Dr. Hughlings Jackson.) Case under the care of HJ.	*Br Med J*, 1872, **ii**: 67–68 20 July 72
72–13 T72 B70	The London Hospital. Sequel of a case of supposed tumour of the middle lobe of the cerebellum (Under the care of Dr. Hughlings Jackson.) Case under the care of HJ.	*Br Med J*, 1872, **ii**: 125 3 Aug 72
72–14 T72 B71	On auditory vertigo (Ménière's disease) By-line.	*Med Times Gaz*, 1872, **ii**: 169–170 17 Aug 72
72–15 T72 B75	London Hospital. A series of cases illustrative of cerebral pathology. Cases of intra-cranial tumour (Under the care of Dr. Hughlings-Jackson) Case under the care of HJ.	*Med Times Gaz*, 1872, **ii**: 541–542 16 Nov 72
72–16 T72 B75	London Hospital. A series of cases illustrative of cerebral pathology. Cases of intra-cranial tumour (Under the care of Dr. Hughlings-Jackson) Case under the care of HJ.	*Med Times Gaz*, 1872, **ii**: 568–569 23 Nov 72

ID	TITLE	PERIODICAL SOURCE
72–17 T72 B75	London Hospital. A series of cases illustrative of cerebral pathology. Cases of intra-cranial tumour (Under the care of Dr. Hughlings-Jackson) Case under the care of HJ.	*Med Times Gaz*, 1872, **ii**: 597–599 30 Nov 72
72–18 T72	On a case of paralysis of the tongue from haemorrhage in the medulla oblongata By-line, with pathology by J Lockhart Clarke.	*Lancet*, 1872, **ii**: 770–773 30 Nov 72
72–19 T72 B75	London Hospital. A series of cases illustrative of cerebral pathology. Cases of intra-cranial tumour (Under the care of Dr. Hughlings-Jackson) Case under the care of HJ.	*Med Times Gaz*, 1872, **ii**: 625–626 7 Dec 72
72–20 T72 B75	London Hospital. A series of cases illustrative of cerebral pathology. Cases of intra-cranial tumour (Under the care of Dr. Hughlings-Jackson) Cases under the care of HJ.	*Med Times Gaz*, 1872, **ii**: 698–699 28 Dec 72

1873

ID	TITLE	PERIODICAL SOURCE
73–01 T73 B76 SW1, pp. 37–76	On the anatomical and physiological localisation of movements in the brain By-line.	*Lancet*, 1873, i: 84–85 18 Jan 73
73–02 T73	On palsy of vocal cord from intracranial syphilis By-line.	*Br Med J*, 1873, i: 86 25 Jan 73
73–03 T73 B76 SW1, pp. 37–76	On the anatomical and physiological localisation of movements in the brain By-line.	*Lancet*, 1873, i: 162–164 1 Feb 72
73–04 T73 B76 SW1, pp. 37–76	On the anatomical and physiological localisation of movements in the brain By-line.	*Lancet*, 1873, i: 232–234 15 Feb 73
73–05 T73	Observations on defects of sight in diseases of the nervous system By-line.	*Royal London Ophthalmic Hospital Reports*, 1873, **7**: 513–527 Issue dated Feb 73
73–06 T73 B75	London Hospital. A series of cases illustrative of cerebral pathology. Cases of intra-cranial tumour (Under the care of Dr. Hughlings-Jackson) Case under the care of HJ.	*Med Times Gaz*, 1873, i: 223–225 1 Mar 73

ID	TITLE	PERIODICAL SOURCE
73–07 T72 B75	London Hospital. A series of cases illustrative of cerebral pathology. Cases of intra-cranial tumour (Under the care of Dr. Hughlings-Jackson) Case under the care of HJ.	*Med Times Gaz*, 1873, **i**: 329–330 29 Mar 73
73–08	London Hospital. Abscess in the left lobe of the cerebellum from suppurative disease of the ear; double optic neuritis (Under the care of Mr. Maunder) Case report contains direct quotation from HJ.	*Lancet*, 1873, **i**: 443–444 29 Mar 73
73–09	Abscess in the right lobe of the cerebellum from aural disease: no optic neuritis (Under the care of Dr. Hughlings Jackson) Case under the care of HJ.	*Lancet*, 1873, **i**: 444–445 29 Mar 73
73–10 T73 B75	London Hospital. A series of cases illustrative of cerebral pathology. Cases of intra-cranial tumour (Under the care of Dr. Hughlings-Jackson) Case under the care of HJ.	*Med Times Gaz*, 1873, **i**: 493–495 10 May 73
73–11 T73 B78 SW1, pp. 112–117	On the anatomical investigation of epilepsy and epileptiform convulsions By-line.	*Br Med J*, 1873, **i**: 531–533 10 May 73
73–12 T73	London Hospital. Notes on cases of disease of the nervous system By-line.	*Br Med J*, 1873, **i**: 560–561 17 May 73
73–13 T73 B75	London Hospital. A series of cases illustrative of cerebral pathology. Cases of intra-cranial tumour (Under the care of Dr. Hughlings-Jackson) Case under the care of HJ.	*Med Times Gaz*, 1873, **ii**: 33–35 12 July 73

ID	TITLE	PERIODICAL SOURCE
73–14 T73	Remarks on the double condition of loss of consciousness and mental automatism following certain epileptic seizures By-line.	*Med Times Gaz*, 1873, **ii**: 63–64 19 July 73
73–15 T73 SW2, pp. 270–286	Lectures on diagnosis of tumours of the brain By-line.	*Med Times Gaz*, 1873, **ii**: 139–140 9 Aug 73
73–16	Forty-first meeting of the British Medical Association. Demonstrations on patients. Report of case presentation by HJ.	*Br Med J*, 1873, **ii**: 239–240 23 Aug 73
73–17 T73 SW2, pp. 270–286	Lectures on diagnosis of tumours of the brain By-line.	*Med Times Gaz*, 1873, **ii**: 195–197 23 Aug 73
73–18 T73	On a case of local softening of the brain from thrombosis of syphilitic arteries By-line.	*Br Med J*, 1873, **ii**: 254 30 Aug 73
73–19 T73 B79	London Hospital. Remarks on cases of vertigo, reeling, and vomiting, from ear disease By-line.	*Lancet*, 1873, **ii**: 334–335 6 Sept 73
73–20 T73	On hemiplegia, with paralysis of the third nerve By-line.	*Lancet*, 1873, **ii**: 335 6 Sept 73
73–21 T73	Pulmonary apoplexies (haemorrhagic infarctions) in cases of cerebral apoplexy By-line.	*Br Med J*, 1873, **ii**: 483–484 25 Oct 73

ID	TITLE	PERIODICAL SOURCE
73–22 T73 SW2, pp. 270–286	Lectures on diagnosis of tumours of the brain By-line.	*Med Times Gaz*, 1873, **ii**: 541–543 15 Nov 73
73–23 T73	London Hospital. Remarks on limited convulsive seizures, and on the after-effects of strong nervous discharges By-line.	*Lancet*, 1873, **ii**: 840–841 13 Dec 73
73–24 T73 B77 SW1, pp. 77–89	Observations on the localisation of movements in the cerebral hemispheres, as revealed by cases of convulsion, chorea and "aphasia" By-line.	*West Riding Lunatic Asylum Medical Reports*, 1873, **3**: 175–195 Volume dated 1873
73–25 T73 B78 SW1, pp. 90–111	On the anatomical, physiological, and pathological investigations of epilepsies By-line.	*West Riding Lunatic Asylum Medical Reports*, 1873, **3**: 315–349 Volume dated 1873

1874

ID	TITLE	PERIODICAL SOURCE
74–01 T74 B75	Hospital for the Epileptic and Paralysed. A series of cases illustrative of cerebral pathology. Cases of intra-cranial tumour (Under the care of Dr. Hughlings-Jackson) Case under the care of HJ.	*Med Times Gaz*, 1874, **i**: 6–7 3 Jan 74
74–02 T74 B91 SW2, pp. 129–145	On the nature of the duality of the brain By-line.	*Med Press Circular*, 1874, **17**: 19–21 14 Jan 74
74–03 T74 B91 SW2, pp. 129–145	On the nature of the duality of the brain By-line.	*Med Press Circular*, 1874, **17**: 41–44 21 Jan 74
74–04 T74 B75	Hospital for the Epileptic and Paralysed. A series of cases illustrative of cerebral pathology. Cases of intra-cranial tumour (Under the care of Dr. Hughlings-Jackson) Case under the care of HJ.	*Med Times Gaz*, 1874, **i**: 96 24 Jan 74
74–05 T74 B91 SW2, pp. 129–145	On the nature of the duality of the brain By-line.	*Med Press Circular*, 1874, **17**: 63–65 28 Jan 74
74–06 T74 B80, B75	London Hospital. A series of cases illustrative of cerebral pathology. Cases of intra-cranial tumour (Under the care of Dr. Hughlings-Jackson) Case under the care of HJ.	*Med Times Gaz*, 1874, **i**: 151–153 7 Feb 74

ID	TITLE	PERIODICAL SOURCE
74–07 T74	Ophthalmoscopic examination during an attack of epileptiform amaurosis By-line.	*Lancet*, 1874, **i**: 193–194 7 Feb 74
74–08 T74 B82	Hospital for the Epileptic and Paralysed. Remarks on coloured vision preceding epileptic seizures By-line.	*Br Med J*, 1874, **i**: 174 7 Feb 74
74–09 B81	Hospital for the Epileptic and Paralysed. On the after-effects of severe epileptic discharges: speculations as to epileptic mania By-line.	*Br Med J*, 1874, **i**: 174 7 Feb 74
74–10 T74 B83 SW1, p. 118	Hospital for the Epileptic and Paralysed. Remarks on systemic sensations in epilepsies By-line.	*Br Med J*, 1874, **i**: 174 7 Feb 74
74–11 T74 B75	London Hospital. A series of cases illustrative of cerebral pathology. Cases of intra-cranial tumour (Under the care of Dr. Hughlings-Jackson) Case under the care of HJ.	*Med Times Gaz*, 1874, **i**: 234–235 24 Feb 74
74–12 T74 B92	Charcot and others on auditory vertigo (Ménière's disease) By-line.	*London Med Record*, 1874, **2**: 238–240 22 Apr 74
74–13 T74 B92	Charcot and others on auditory vertigo (Ménière's disease) By-line.	*London Med Record*, 1874, **2**: 254–256 29 Apr 74
74–14 T74 B84	Temporary affection of speech (aphasia): "aphasic" writing By-line.	*Br Med J*, 1874, **i**: 574 2 May 74

ID	TITLE	PERIODICAL SOURCE
74–15	London Hospital. On a case of recovery from hemiplegia (Under the care of Dr. Hughlings Jackson) Case under the care of HJ.	*Lancet*, 1874, **i**: 618–619 2 May 74
74–16 T74	The comparative study of drunkenness Unsigned editorial, claimed in first person singular in *Med Press Circular*, 1881, **31**: 329–332, on p. 330n.	*Br Med J*, 1874, **i**: 652–653 16 May 74
74–17 T74	The comparative study of drunkenness Unsigned editorial, claimed in first person singular in *Med Press Circular*, 1881, **31**: 329–332, on p. 330n	*Br Med J*, 1874, **i**: 685–686 23 May 74
74–18 T74 B85	A case of right hemiplegia and loss of speech from local softening of the brain By-line.	*Br Med J*, 1874, **i**: 804–805 20 June 74
74–19 T74 B85	Clinical lecture on a case of hemiplegia By-line.	*Br Med J*, 1874, **ii**: 69–71 18 July 74
74–20 T74 B86	Clinical lecture on a case of hemiplegia By-line.	*Br Med J*, 1874, **ii**: 99–101 25 July 74
74–21 T74 B90	Two cases of intra-cranial syphilis By-line.	*J Mental Sci*, 1874, **20**: 235–243 Issue dated July 74
74–22 T74 B87	London Hospital. A series of cases illustrative of cerebral pathology. Cases of intracranial tumour (Under the care of Dr. Hughlings-Jackson) Case under the care of HJ.	*Med Times Gaz*, 1874, **ii**: 118–119 1 Aug 74

ID	TITLE	PERIODICAL SOURCE
74–23	Jackson on syphilitic disease within the cranium	*London Med Record*, 1874, **2**: 635–666
	Review by W Bathurst Woodman of pamphlet by HJ.	7 Oct 74
74–24	Jackson on hemiplegia	*London Med Record*, 1874, **2**: 648–650
	Review by W Bathurst Woodman of HJ's published work.	14 Oct 74
74–25 T74 B94 SW1, pp. 162–273	On the scientific and empirical investigation of epilepsies	*Med Press Circular*, 1874, **18**: 325–327
	By-line.	14 Oct 74
74–26 T74 B75	Hospital for the Epileptic and Paralysed. A series of cases illustrative of cerebral pathology. Cases of intra-cranial tumour (Under the care of Dr. Hughlings-Jackson)	*Med Times Gaz*, 1874, **ii**: 441–442
	Case under the care of HJ.	17 Oct 74
74–27 T74 B94 SW1, pp. 162–273	On the scientific and empirical investigation of epilepsies	*Med Press Circular*, 1874, **18**: 347–352
	By-line.	21 Oct 74
74–28 T74 B75	London Hospital. A series of cases illustrative of cerebral pathology. Cases of intra-cranial tumour (Under the care of Dr. Hughlings-Jackson)	*Med Times Gaz*, 1874, **ii**: 471–472
	Case under the care of HJ.	24 Oct 74
74–29 T74 B88	London Hospital. Remarks on loss of smell and taste	*Lancet*, 1874, **ii**: 622
	By-line.	31 Oct 74

ID	TITLE	PERIODICAL SOURCE
74–30	Periscope	*Royal London Ophthalmic Hospital Reports*, 1874, **8**: 88–102
	Review of HJ's published work.	Issue dated Oct 74
74–31 T74 B94 SW1, pp. 162–273	On the scientific and empirical investigation of epilepsies By-line.	*Med Press Circular*, 1874, **18**: 389–392 4 Nov 74
74–32 T74 B94 SW1, pp. 162–273	On the scientific and empirical investigation of epilepsies By-line.	*Med Press Circular*, 1874, **18**: 409–412 11 Nov 74
74–33 T74 B89	London Hospital. Attacks of giddiness and vomiting, with deafness and ear disease (Under the care of Dr. Hughlings Jackson) Case under the care of HJ.	*Lancet*, 1874, **ii**: 727–728 21 Nov 74
74–34 T74 B94 SW1, pp. 162–273	On the scientific and empirical investigation of epilepsies By-line.	*Med Press Circular*, 1874, **18**: 475–478 2 Dec 74
74–35 T74 B94 SW1, pp. 162–273	On the scientific and empirical investigation of epilepsies By-line.	*Med Press Circular*, 1874, **18**: 497–499 9 Dec 74
74–36 T74 B94 SW1, pp. 162–273	On the scientific and empirical investigation of epilepsies By-line.	*Med Press Circular*, 1874, **18**: 519–521 16 Dec 74

ID	TITLE	PERIODICAL SOURCE
74–37 B73	On a case of recovery from hemiplegia. Much damage of motor tract and convolutions remaining. Remarks on chorea By-line.	*St Andrews Medical Graduates' Association Transactions 1872 and 1873*, 60–68 Volume dated 1874
74–38 T74 B93	On a case of recovery from double optic neuritis By-line.	*West Riding Lunatic Asylum Medical Reports*, 1874, **4**: 24–29 Volume dated 1874

1875

ID	TITLE	PERIODICAL SOURCE
75–01 T75 B96	London Hospital. Clinical observations on cases of disease of the nervous system By-line.	*Lancet*, 1875, **i**: 85 16 Jan 75
75–02 T75 B97 B98	London Hospital. Cases of nervous disease; with clinical remarks (Under the care of Dr. Hughlings Jackson) Case under the care of HJ.	*Lancet*, 1875, **i**: 161 30 Jan 75
75–03 T75 B95	Nervous symptoms in cases of congenital syphilis By-line.	*J Mental Sci*, 1875, **20**: 517–527 Issue dated Jan 75
75–04 T75 B94 SW1, pp. 162–273	On the scientific and empirical investigation of epilepsies By-line.	*Med Press Circular*, 1875, **19**: 353–355 26 Apr 75
75–05 T75 B75	London Hospital. Cases illustrative of cerebral pathology. Cases of intracranial tumour (Under the care of Dr. Hughlings-Jackson) Case under the care of HJ.	*Med Times Gaz*, 1875, **i**: 468–469 1 May 75
75–06 T75	London Hospital. Remarks on difficulties in the diagnosis of causes of apoplexy By-line.	*Med Times Gaz*, 1875, **i**: 498–499 8 May 75
75–07 T75 B94 SW1, pp. 162–273	On the scientific and empirical investigation of epilepsies By-line.	*Med Press Circular*, 1875, **19**: 397–400 12 May 75

ID	TITLE	PERIODICAL SOURCE
75–08 T75 B99	On choreal movements and cerebellar rigidity in a case of tubercular meningitis By-line.	*Br Med J*, 1875, i: 636–637 15 May 75
75–09 T75	On automatic actions during coma from cerebral haemorrhage By-line.	*Med Times Gaz*, 1875, i: 522 15 May 75
75–10 T75 B94 SW1, pp. 162–273	On the scientific and empirical investigation of epilepsies By-line.	*Med Press Circular*, 1875, **19**: 419–421 19 May 75
75–11 T75 B100	Hospital for the Epileptic and Paralysed. Autopsy on a case of hemiopia with hemiplegia and hemianaesthesia By-line.	*Lancet*, 1875, i: 722 22 May 75
75–12	Hospital for the Epileptic and Paralysed. Remarks on cases of hemiopsia with hemiplegia By-line.	*Lancet*, 1875, i: 722 22 May 75
75–13 T75 B102	London Hospital. Cases of partial convulsion from organic brain disease, bearing on the experiments of Hitzig and Ferrier By-line.	*Med Times Gaz*, 1875, i: 578–579 29 May 75
75–14 T75 B102	London Hospital. Cases of partial convulsion from organic brain disease, bearing on the experiments of Hitzig and Ferrier By-line.	*Med Times Gaz*, 1875, i: 606–607 5 June 75

ID	TITLE	PERIODICAL SOURCE
75–15	Hughlings Jackson on nervous dissolution, as illustrated by epileptic mania	*London Med Record*, 1875, **3**: 349–350
	Report of HJ's published views.	Issue dated 9 June 75
75–16 T75 B101	London Hospital. Clinical memoranda of a series of interesting cases of nerve-disorder now in hospital (Under the care of Dr. Hughlings Jackson)	*Br Med J*, 1875, **i**: 773–774
	Case under the care of HJ.	12 June 75
75–17	Hughlings Jackson on cases of nervous disease	*London Med Record* 1875, **3**: 367–368
	Report of HJ's published views.	Issue dated 16 June 75
75–18	On nervous dissolution	*London Med Record*, 1875, **3**: 790–380
	By-lined letter.	Issue dated 16 June 75
75–19 T75 B102	London Hospital. Cases of partial convulsion from organic brain disease, bearing on the experiments of Hitzig and Ferrier	*Med Times Gaz*, 1875, **i**: 660–661
	By-line.	19 June 75
75–20	Hughlings Jackson on difficulties in the diagnosis of the causes of apoplexy	*London Med Record*, 1875, **3**: 398–399
	By-line.	30 June 75
75–21	Hemikinesis	*Br Med J*, 1875, **ii**: 43
	By-lined letter.	10 July 75

ID	TITLE	PERIODICAL SOURCE
75–22 T75 B102	London Hospital. Cases of partial convulsion from organic brain disease, bearing on the experiments of Hitzig and Ferrier By-line.	*Med Times Gaz*, 1875, **ii**: 94 24 July 75
75–23 T75	On a case of nearly complete deafness following apoplexy By-line.	*Med Times Gaz*, 1875, **ii**: 118 31 July 75
75–24 T75 B106 SW2, pp. 287–299	On syphilitic affections of the nervous system By-line.	*J Mental Sci*, 1875, **20**: 207–225 Issue dated July 75
75–25 T75	The London Hospital. Observations of Ménière's disease Report of HJ's views.	*Med Times Gaz*, 1875, **ii**: 161–162 7 Aug 75
75–26 T75 B103	Hospital for the Paralysed and Epileptic. Case illustrating the relation betwixt certain cases of migraine and epilepsy By-line.	*Lancet*, 1875, **ii**: 244–245 14 Aug 75
75–27 T75 B102	The London Hospital. Cases of partial convulsion from organic brain disease, bearing on experiments of Hitzig and Ferrier By-line.	*Med Times Gaz*, 1875, **ii**: 264–266 4 Sept 75
75–28 T75 B104	A lecture on softening of the brain By-line.	*Lancet*, 1875, **ii**: 335–339 4 Sept 75

ID	TITLE	PERIODICAL SOURCE
75–29 T75 B102	The London Hospital. Cases of partial convulsion from organic brain disease, bearing on experiments of Hitzig and Ferrier By-line.	*Med Times Gaz*, 1875, **ii**: 330–331 18 Sept 75
75–30 T75	A periscope of contemporary ophthalmic literature Report of HJ's published views.	*Royal London Ophthalmic Hospital Reports*, 1875, **8**: 318–343 Issue dated Sept 75
75–31 T75	Editorial comment Editorial report of HJ's views.	*Lancet*, 1875, **ii**: 497–498 2 Oct 75
75–32 T75 B94 SW1, pp. 162–273	On the scientific and empirical investigation of epilepsies By-line.	*Med Press Circular*, 1875, **20**: 313–315 20 Oct 75
75–33 T75	Royal Medical and Chirurgical Society. On the pathology of chorea Report of HJ's views.	*Med Times Gaz*, 1875, **ii**: 481–483 23 Oct 75
75–34 T75 B94 SW1, pp. 162–273	On the scientific and empirical investigation of epilepsies By-line.	*Med Press Circular*, 1875, **20**: 355–358 3 Nov 75
75–35 T75 B94 SW1, pp. 162–273	On the scientific and empirical investigation of epilepsies By-line.	*Med Press Circular*, 1875, **20**: 487–489 15 Dec 75

ID	TITLE	PERIODICAL SOURCE
75–36 T75 B105 SW1, pp. 119–134	On temporary mental disorders after epileptic paroxysms By-line.	*West Riding Lunatic Asylum Medical Reports*, 1875, **5**: 105–129 Volume dated 1875

1876

ID	TITLE	PERIODICAL SOURCE
76–01 T75 B102	The London Hospital. Cases of partial convulsion from organic brain disease, bearing on experiments of Hitzig and Ferrier By-line.	*Med Times Gaz*, 1876, **i**: 8–10 1 Jan 76
76–02	Jackson on temporary mental disorders after epileptic paroxysms Review by H Sunderland of HJ's views.	*London Med Record*, 1876, **4**: 22–23 15 Jan 76
76–03	Clinical and physiological researches on the nervous system. No. 1 Unsigned review of HJ's pamphlet.	*London Med Record*, 1876, **4**: 43–44 15 Jan 76
76–04 T76 B94 SW1, pp. 162–273	On the scientific and empirical investigation of epilepsies By-line.	*Med Press Circular*, 1876, **21**: 63–65 26 Jan 76
76–05 T76 B94 SW1, pp. 162–273	On the scientific and empirical investigation of epilepsies By-line.	*Med Press Circular*, 1876, **21**: 129–131 16 Feb 76
76–06 T76 B109	Les troubles intellectuels momentanées qui suivant les accès épileptiques By-line.	*Revue Scientifique de la France et de l'Etranger*, 1876, 2nd series, 5th year, no. 34: 169–178 19 Feb 76

ID	TITLE	PERIODICAL SOURCE
76–07 T76 B94 SW1, pp. 162–273	On the scientific and empirical investigation of epilepsies By-line.	*Med Press Circular*, 1876, **21**: 173–176 1 Mar 76
76–08 T76	Notes on cases of disease of the nervous system By-line.	*Med Examiner*, 1876, **1**: 170–171 2 Mar 76
76–09 T76 B107	Hospital for the Epileptic and Paralysed. On cases of epileptic seizures, with an auditory warning. By-line.	*Lancet*, 1876, **i**: 386–387 11 Mar 76
76–10 T76	The London Hospital. Epilepsy—automatic and unconscious performance of complex actions in epilepsy (Under the care of Dr. Hughlings-Jackson. Reported by Mr. R. Atkinson) Case under the care of HJ, reported by R Atkinson.	*Med Times Gaz*, 1876, **i**: 304 18 Mar 76
76–11 T76 B94 SW1, pp. 162–273	On the scientific and empirical investigation of epilepsies By-line.	*Med Press Circular*, 1876, **21**: 313–316 19 Apr 76
76–12 T76 SW2, pp. 146–152	Case of large cerebral tumour without optic neuritis and with left hemiplegia and imperception By-line.	*Royal London Ophthalmic Hospital Reports*, 1876, **8**: 434–444 Issue dated May 76

ID	TITLE	PERIODICAL SOURCE
76–13 T76	A case of double optic neuritis without cerebral tumour By-line.	*Royal London Ophthalmic Hospital Reports*, 1876, **8**: 445–455 Issue dated May 76
76–14 B94 SW1, pp. 162–273	On the scientific and empirical investigation of epilepsies By-line.	*Med Press Circular*, 1876, **21**: 479–481 14 June 76
76–15 T76 B94 SW1, pp. 162–273	On the scientific and empirical investigation of epilepsies By-line.	*Med Press Circular*, 1876, **22**: 145–147 23 Aug 76
76–16 T76 B94 SW1, pp. 162–273	On the scientific and empirical investigation of epilepsies By-line.	*Med Press Circular*, 1876, **22**: 185–187 6 Sept 76
76–17 T76 B112	Clinical and physiological researches on the nervous system Third person review.	*J Psychol Med Mental Pathol*, 1876, n.s. **2** (1): 150–155 Before Oct 76
76–18 T76 B94 SW1, pp. 162–273	On the scientific and empirical investigation of epilepsies By-line.	*Med Press Circular*, 1876, **22**: 475–477 13 Dec 76

ID	TITLE	PERIODICAL SOURCE
76–19 T76	On the gravity of cerebral lesions By-line.	*Med Examiner*, 1876, **2**: 890–891 21 Dec 76
76–20 T76 B110	Note on the "embolic theory" of chorea By-line.	*Br Med J*, 1876, **ii**: 813–814 23 Dec 76
76–21 T76 B108 SW1, pp. 274–275	London Hospital. Notes on cases of disease of the nervous system (Under the care of Dr. Hughlings-Jackson) Case under the care of HJ.	*Med Times Gaz*, 1876, **ii**: 700–702 23 Dec 76
76–22 T76 B111 SW1, pp. 135–161	On epilepsies and on the after-effects of epileptic discharges (Todd and Robertson's hypothesis) By-line.	*West Riding Lunatic Asylum Medical Reports*, 1876, **6**: 266–309 Volume printed 1876

1877

ID	TITLE	PERIODICAL SOURCE
77–01 T77	On nervous symptoms with ear disease By-line.	*Lancet*, 1877, **i**: 415–417 24 Mar 77
77–02 T77	On nervous symptoms with ear disease By-line.	*Br Med J*, 1877, **i**: 349–351 24 Mar 77
77–03	On nervous symptoms with ear disease By-line.	*Med Times Gaz*, 1877, **i**: 308–310 24 Mar 77
77–04 T77 B113	London Hospital. Cases of tumour of the middle lobe of the cerebellum (Under the care of Dr. Hughlings Jackson) Case under the care of HJ.	*Br Med J*, 1877, **i**: 354 24 Mar 77
77–05 T77 B114	London Hospital. Hemiplegia coming on without loss of consciousness; death; autopsy; atheromatous and syphilitic disease of cerebral arteries (Under the care of Dr. Hughlings Jackson) Case under the care of HJ.	*Lancet*, 1877, **i**: 457–458 31 Mar 77
77–06	On unconscious and automatic actions after epileptic fits. 1 Unsigned editorial, claimed in first person singular in *Med Press Circular*, 1881, **31**: 329–332, on p. 330n.	*Br Med J*, 1877, **i**: 393–395 31 Mar 77
77–07 T77 B116	Remarks on rigidity in hemiplegia By-line.	*Med Examiner*, 1877, **2**: 271–272 5 Apr 77

ID	TITLE	PERIODICAL SOURCE
77–08	On unconscious and automatic actions after epileptic fits. 2 Unsigned editorial, claimed in first person singular in *Med Press Circular* 1881, **31**: 329–332, on p. 330n.	*Br Med J*, 1877, **i**: 431–432 7 Apr 77
77–09 T77 SW2, pp. 300–319	Ophthalmology in its relation to general medicine By-line.	*Med Examiner*, 1877, **2**: 365–367 10 May 77
77–10 T77 SW2, pp. 300–319	An address on ophthalmology in its relation to general medicine By-line.	*Br Med J*, 1877, **i**: 575–577 12 May 77
77–11 SW2, pp. 300–319	Ophthalmology in its relation to general medicine By-line.	*Lancet*, 1877, **i**: 674–678 12 May 77
77–12 T77 SW2, pp. 300–319	Ophthalmology in its relation to general medicine By-line.	*Med Times Gaz*, 1877, **i**: 496–500 12 May 77
77–13 T77 SW2, pp. 300–319	Ophthalmology in its relation to general medicine By-line.	*Med Examiner*, 1877, **2**: 388–390 17 May 77
77–14 T77 SW2, pp. 300–319	An address on ophthalmology in its relation to general medicine By-line.	*Br Med J*, 1877, **i**: 605–606 19 May 77
77–15 T77 SW2, pp. 300–319	Ophthalmology in its relation to general medicine By-line.	*Med Examiner*, 1877, **2**: 427–429 31 May 77
77–16 T77 SW2, pp. 300–319	An address on ophthalmology in its relation to general medicine By-line.	*Br Med J*, 1877, **i**: 672–674 2 June 77

ID	TITLE	PERIODICAL SOURCE
77–17 T77 SW2, pp. 300–319	Ophthalmology in its relation to general medicine By-line.	*Med Examiner*, 1877, **2**: 448–40 7 June 77
77–18 T77 SW2, pp. 300–319	An address on ophthalmology in its relation to general medicine By-line.	*Br Med J*, 1877, **i**: 703–705 9 June 77
77–19 T77 SW2, pp. 300–319	Ophthalmology in its relation to general medicine By-line.	*Med Examiner*, 1877, **2**: 467–468 14 June 77
77–20 T77 B115	London Hospital. Case of suspected "discharging lesion" of the hinder part of the uppermost right frontal convolution—illustration of Ferrier's researches (Under the care of Dr. Hughlings Jackson) Case under the care of HJ.	*Lancet*, 1877, **i**: 876 16 June 77
77–21 T77 SW2, pp. 300–319	Ophthalmology in its relation to general medicine By-line.	*Med Examiner*, 1877, **2**: 509–510 28 June 77
77–22 T77 SW2, pp. 300–319	An address on ophthalmology in its relation to general medicine By-line.	*Br Med J*, 1877, **i**: 804–805 30 June 77
77–23 T77	Clinical notes on nervous disease: case of convulsions from syphilitic disease of the brain By-line.	*Med Examiner*, 1877, **2**: 1018–1019 13 Dec 77

1878

ID	TITLE	PERIODICAL SOURCE
78–01 T78 B117	On cerebral paresis or paralysis with cerebellar tremor or rigidity By-line.	*Med Examiner*, 1878, **3**: 266–277 28 Mar 78
78–02 T78 B118 SW2, pp. 153–154	London Hospital. Remarks on non-protrusion of the tongue in some cases of aphasia By-line.	*Lancet*, 1878, **i**: 716–717 18 May 78
78–03	Buzzard on blepharospasm By-line.	*Brain*, 1878, **1**: 285–286 Issue dated July 78
78–04 T78	Remarks on comparison and contrast betwixt tetanus and a certain epileptiform seizure By-line.	*Med Times Gaz*, 1878, **ii**: 484–485 26 Oct 78
78–05 T78 B119	Remarks on the cerebellum By-line.	*Med Times Gaz*, 1878, **ii**: 485–486 26 Oct 78
78–06 T78 B120	London Hospital. Case of temporary hemiplegia after localised epileptiform convulsion (Under the care of Dr. Hughlings Jackson) Case under the care of HJ.	*Lancet*, 1878, **ii**: 581–582 26 Oct 78
78–07 T78 SW2, pp. 155–183	On affections of speech from disease of the brain By-line.	*Brain*, 1878, **1**: 304–330 Issue dated Oct 78

ID	TITLE	PERIODICAL SOURCE
78–08 T78 B120a	London Hospital. Tetanus-like seizures with double optic neuritis—no autopsy (Under the care of Dr. Hughlings-Jackson) Case under the care of HJ.	*Med Times Gaz*, 1878, **ii**: 596–597 23 Nov 78

1879

ID	TITLE	PERIODICAL SOURCE
79–01 T79 B121 SW1, pp. 276–307	Lectures on the diagnosis of epilepsy By-line.	*Med Times Gaz*, 1879, **i**: 29–33 11 Jan 79
79–02 B121	Abstract of lectures on the diagnosis of epilepsy By-line.	*Lancet*, 1879, **i**: 42–43 11 Jan 79
79–03 B121	Lectures on the diagnosis of epilepsy. Delivered before the Harveian Society By-line.	*Br Med J*, 1879, **i**: 33–36 11 Jan 79
79–04 T79 B121 SW1, pp. 276–307	Lectures on the diagnosis of epilepsy By-line.	*Med Times Gaz*, 1879, **i**: 85–88 25 Jan 79
79–05 B121	Abstract of lectures on the diagnosis of epilepsy By-line.	*Lancet*, 1879, **i**: 110–112 25 Jan 79
79–06 B121	Lectures on the diagnosis of epilepsy. Delivered before the Harveian Society By-line.	*Br Med J*, 1879, **i**: 109–112 25 Jan 79
79–07 B121 SW1, pp. 276–307	Lectures on the diagnosis of epilepsy. Delivered before the Harveian Society By-line.	*Br Med J*, 1879, **i**: 141–143 1 Feb 79
79–08 T79 B121 SW1, pp. 276–307	Lectures on the diagnosis of epilepsy By-line.	*Med Times Gaz*, 1879, **i**: 141–143 8 Feb 79

ID	TITLE	PERIODICAL SOURCE
79–09 B121	Abstract of lectures on the diagnosis of epilepsy By-line.	*Lancet*, 1879, **i**: 184–185 8 Feb 79
79–10 T79 B121 SW1, pp. 276–307	Lectures on the diagnosis of epilepsy By-line.	*Med Times Gaz*, 1879, **i**: 223–226 1 Mar 79
79–11 T79 B123	Auditory vertigo By-line.	*Brain*, 1879, **2**: 29–38 Issue of Apr 79
79–12 T79 B122	Remarks on the routine use of the ophthalmoscope in cerebral disease By-line.	*Med Press Circular*, 1879, **27**: 439–441 4 June 79
79–13 T79 B122	Remarks on the routine use of the ophthalmoscope in cerebral disease By-line.	*Med Press Circular*, 1879, **27**: 459–461 11 June 79
79–14 T79 B122	Remarks on the routine use of the ophthalmoscope in cerebral disease By-line.	*Med Press Circular*, 1879, **27**: 479–480 18 June 79
79–15 T79 SW2, pp. 171–183	On affections of speech from disease of the brain By-line.	*Brain*, 1879, **2**: 203–222 Issue dated July 79
79–16	Note on Dr. J. Hughlings-Jackson's case of auditory vertigo in April no. of *Brain* letter from J Taylor with by-lined response from HJ.	*Brain*, 1879, **2**: 273–274 Issue dated July 79

ID	TITLE	PERIODICAL SOURCE
79–17 T79	Psychology and the nervous system	*Med Press Circular*, 1879, **28**: 199–201
	By-line.	3 Sept 79
79–18 T79	Psychology and the nervous system	*Med Press Circular*, 1879, **28**: 239–241
	By-line.	17 Sept 79
79–19 T79	Psychology and the nervous system	*Med Press Circular*, 1879, **28**: 283–285
	By-line.	1 Oct 79
79–20 T79 SW2, pp. 184–204	On affections of speech from disease of the brain	*Brain*, 1879, **2**: 323–356
	By-line.	Issue dated Oct 79
79–21 T79	Psychology and the nervous system	*Med Press Circular*, 1879, **28**: 409–411
	By-line.	12 Nov 79
79–22 T79	Psychology and the nervous system	*Med Press Circular*, 1879, **28**: 429–430
	By-line.	19 Nov 79

1880

ID	TITLE	PERIODICAL SOURCE
80–01 T80	On tumours of the cerebellum	*Lancet*, 1880, **i**: 122–124
	By-line.	24 Jan 80
80–02 T80	Remarks on tumours of the cerebellum	*Br Med J*, 1880, **i**: 196–198
	By-line.	7 Feb 80
80–03 T80	Lecture on a case of intracranial syphilis	*Lancet*, 1880, **i**: 275–277
	By-line.	21 Feb 80
80–04 T80	Lecture on a case of intracranial syphilis	*Lancet*, 1880, **i**: 357–359
	By-line.	6 Mar 80
80–05 T80	On affections of speech	*Med Press Circular*, 1880, **29**: 253–255
	By-line.	31 Mar 80
80–06 T80 B124	On aphasia, with left hemiplegia	*Lancet*, 1880, **i**: 637–638
	By-line.	24 Apr 80
80–07 T80	Remarks on diseases of the cerebellum	*Med Press Circular*, 1880, **29**: 448–449
	By-line.	2 June 80
80–08 T80	Remarks on diseases of the cerebellum	*Med Press Circular*, 1880, **29**: 469–471
	By-line.	9 June 80

ID	TITLE	PERIODICAL SOURCE
80–09 T80	Case illustrating the value of the ophthalmoscope in the investigation and treatment of diseases of the brain By-line.	*Lancet*, 1880, **i**: 906 12 June 80
80–10 T80 SW1, pp. 308–317	On right or left-sided spasm at the onset of epileptic paroxysms, and on crude sensation warnings and elaborate mental states By-line.	*Brain*, 1880, **3**: 192–206 Issue dated July 80
80–11	Buzzard on certain points in tabes dorsalis By-line.	*Brain*, 1880, **3**: 266–268 Issue dated July 80
80–12 T80 B125 SW2, pp. 320–327	Part of a lecture on auditory vertigo By-line.	*Lancet*, 1880, **ii**: 525–528 2 Oct 80
80–13 T80 B126	On a case of recovery from organic brain-disease By-line.	*Br Med J*, 1880, **ii**: 654–656 23 Oct 80
80–14 T80	National Hospital for the Epileptic and Paralysed. Peculiar phenomena after epileptic seizures (Under the care of Dr. Hughlings Jackson) Case under the care of HJ.	*Br Med J*, 1880, **ii**: 776–777 13 Nov 80
80–15 T80	Eye symptoms in locomotor ataxy By-line.	*Lancet*, 1880, **ii**: 968–969 18 Dec 80
80–16	Ophthalmological Society of the United Kingdom. Eye-symptoms in locomotor ataxy Report of paper read by HJ.	*Br Med J*, 1880, **ii**: 980–981 18 Dec 80

1881

ID	TITLE	PERIODICAL SOURCE
81–01 T81 B128	On a case of temporary left hemiplegia, with foot-clonus and exaggerated knee-phenomenon, after an epileptiform seizure beginning in the left foot By-line.	*Med Times Gaz*, 1881, **i**: 183–186 12 Jan 81
81–02 T80 B127 SW1, pp. 318–329	On temporary paralysis after epileptiform and epileptic seizures; a contribution to the study of dissolution of the nervous system By-line.	*Brain*, 1881, **3**: 433–451 Issue dated Jan 81
81–03	Buzzard on transfer-phenomena in epilepsy produced by encircling blisters By-line.	*Brain*, 1881, **3**: 554–555 Issue dated Jan 81
81–04 T81 B129	Harveian Society of London. A case of temporary hemiplegia after localised convulsion Report of paper read by HJ.	*Lancet*, 1881, **i**: 335 26 Feb 81
81–05 T81 B130	On optic neuritis in intracranial disease By-line.	*Med Times Gaz*, 1881, **i**: 311–317 19 Mar 81
81–06 T81	Ophthalmological Society of Great Britain [*sic*]. Optic neuritis in intracranial disease Report of remarks by HJ.	*Br Med J*, 1881, **i**: 472–474 26 Mar 81
81–07 T81	Ophthalmological Society Report of case presentation by HJ on optic neuritis.	*Med Times Gaz*, 1881, **i**: 434 16 Apr 81

ID	TITLE	PERIODICAL SOURCE
81–08 T81 B133 SW2, pp. 3–28	Remarks on dissolution of the nervous system, as exemplified by certain post-epileptic conditions By-line.	*Med Press Circular*, 1881, **31**: 329–332 20 Apr 81
81–09	The discussion on optic neuritis at the ophthalmological society Report of discussion by HJ.	*Med Times Gaz*, 1881, **i**: 460–461 23 Apr 81
81–10	Ophthalmological Society of Great Britain [*sic*]. Case illustrating the condition of the discs ten years after optic neuritis Report of case presentation by HJ.	*Br Med J*, 1881, **i**: 645–646 23 Apr 81
81–11 T81 B133 SW2, pp. 3–28	Remarks on dissolution of the nervous system, as exemplified by certain post-epileptic conditions By-line.	*Med Press Circular*, 1881, **31**: 399–400 11 May 81
81–12 T81 B133 SW2, pp. 3–28	Remarks on dissolution of the nervous system, as exemplified by certain post-epileptic conditions By-line.	*Med Press Circular*, 1881, **32**: 68–70 27 July 81
81–13	Buzzard on the affection of bones and joints in locomotor ataxy, and its association with gastric crises By-line.	*Brain*, 1881, **4**: 276–278 Issue dated July 81
81–14	Buzzard on acute anterior polio-myelitis in infants and adults By-line.	*Brain*, 1881, **4**: 278–280 Issue dated July 81

ID	TITLE	PERIODICAL SOURCE
81–15	Buzzard on tendon reflex in the diagnosis of diseases of the spinal cord By-line.	*Brain*, 1881, **4**: 280–82 Issue dated July 81
81–16	Epileptiform convulsions from cerebral disease By-line.	*Br Med J*, 1881, **ii**: 322–323 20 Aug 81
81–17	Ophthalmological Society of Great Britain [*sic*]. The relation between the apparent movement of objects and the rotation of the eyes Report of discussion by HJ.	*Br Med J*, 1881, **ii**: 667–668, on p. 667 22 Oct 81
81–18 T81 B133 SW2, pp. 3–28	Remarks on dissolution of the nervous system, as exemplified by certain post-epileptic conditions By-line.	*Med Press Circular*, 1881, **32**: 380–382 2 Nov 81
81–19 T81 B133 SW2, pp. 3–28	Remarks on dissolution of the nervous system, as exemplified by certain post-epileptic conditions By-line.	*Med Press Circular*, 1881, **32**: 399–401 9 Nov 81
81–20 T81 B133 SW2, pp. 3–28	Remarks on dissolution of the nervous system, as exemplified by certain post-epileptic conditions By-line.	*Med Press Circular*, 1881, **32**: 421–422 16 Nov 81
81–21 T81	Discussion on the relation between optic neuritis and intracranial disease By-line.	*Trans Ophthalmol Soc UK*, 1881, **1**: 60–115 Volume printed 1881

ID	TITLE	PERIODICAL SOURCE
81–22 T81 B131	On eye symptoms in locomotor ataxy By-line.	*Trans Ophthalmol Soc UK*, 1881, **1**: 139–154 Volume printed 1881
81–23 T81 B132 SW1, pp. 330–340	Epileptiform convulsions from cerebral disease By-line.	*Trans International Medical Congress, Seventh Session, 1881*, 1881, **2**: 6–15 Volume printed 1881
81–24 T81 SW1, pp. 330–340	Epileptiform convulsions from cerebral disease By-line.	*Trans International Medical Congress, Seventh Session, 1881*, 1881, **2**: 21–22 Volume printed 1881
81–25 T81	Contribution to discussion on connection between optic neuritis and intracranial disease By-line.	*Trans International Medical Congress, Seventh Session, 1881*, 1881, **3**: 61 Volume printed 1881
81–26 T80 B134 SW2, pp. 328–333	On tumours of the cerebellum By-line.	*Proc Med Soc London*, 1880, **5**: 48–56 Edition printed 1881

ID	TITLE	PERIODICAL SOURCE
81–27 T80	A case of recovery from symptoms of brain disease By-line.	*Proc Med Soc London*, 1880, **5**: 175–178 Edition printed 1881

1882

ID	TITLE	PERIODICAL SOURCE
82–01 T82	Medical Society of London. Cortical tumour of brain Report of paper read by HJ.	*Lancet*, 1882, **i**: 441 18 Mar 82
82–02	Epidemiological Society. South-eastern branch: East and West Surrey districts. Observations on migraine Report of discussion by HJ.	*Br Med J*, 1882, **i**: 464 1 Apr 82
82–03 T82 B135 SW2, pp. 334–342	An address delivered at the opening of the section of pathology, at the Annual Meeting of the British Medical Association, in Worcester, August 1882 By-line.	*Br Med J*, 1882, **ii**: 305–308 19 Aug 82
82–04 T82 SW2, pp. 334–342	Address delivered at the opening of the section of pathology, at the Annual Meeting of the British Medical Association, in Worcester, August, 1882 By-line.	*Med Times Gaz*, 1882, **ii**: 239–242 26 Aug 82
82–05	The study of pathology Report of lecture by HJ.	*Br Med J*, 1882, **ii**: 494–495 9 Sept 82
82–06 T82 B138 SW1, pp. 341–347	Localised convulsions from tumour of the brain By-line.	*Brain*, 1882, **5**: 364–374 Issue dated Oct 82
82–07	Buzzard on diseases of the nervous system By-line.	*Brain*, 1882, **5**: 382–388 Issue dated Oct 82

ID	TITLE	PERIODICAL SOURCE
82–08 T82 B136 SW2, pp. 29–44	On some implications of dissolution of the nervous system By-line.	*Med Press Circular*, 1882, **34**: 411–414 15 Nov 82
82–09 T82 B136 SW2, pp. 29–44	On some implications of dissolution of the nervous system By-line.	*Med Press Circular*, 1882, **34**: 433–434 22 Nov 82
82–10	On the relation between the apparent movements of objects and the rotation of the eyes By-line Professor Donders, Utrecht, communicated, with discussion, by HJ.	*Trans Ophthalmol Soc UK*, 1882, **2**: 213–217 Volume printed 1882

1883

ID	TITLE	PERIODICAL SOURCE
83–01	Commentary Third person report.	*Trans Ophthalmol Soc UK*, 1883, **3**: 229–232 Issue dated Jan 83
83–02 T83 B137 SW2, p. 343	On ocular movements, with vertigo, produced by pressure on a diseased ear By-line.	*Trans Ophthalmol Soc UK*, 1883, **3**: 261–265 Issue dated Jan 1883
83–03	Movements of the eyes provoked by pressure on a diseased ear Report of paper read by HJ.	*Br Med J*, 1883, **i**: 113 20 Jan 83
83–04 T83	The Ophthalmological Society. Movements of the eyes provoked by pressure on a diseased ear Report of paper read by HJ.	*Med Times Gaz*, 1883, **i**: 80–81 20 Jan 83
83–05 T83	Ophthalmological Society of the United Kingdom. Eye symptoms in spinal disease Report of case report by Gowers, discussed by HJ.	*Br Med J*, 1883, **i**: 1180–1182 16 June 83
83–06 T83	The Ophthalmological Society. The relation of eye symptoms to diseases of the spinal cord Report of case report by Gowers, discussed by HJ.	*Med Times Gaz*, 1883, **i**: 684–685 16 June 83
83–07 T82 B136	On some implications of dissolution of the nervous system By-line.	*Med Press Circular*, 1883, **36**: 64–66 25 July 83

ID	TITLE	PERIODICAL SOURCE
83–08 T82 B136	On some implications of dissolution of the nervous system By-line.	*Med Press Circular*, 1883, **36**: 84–86 1 Aug 83

1884

ID	TITLE	PERIODICAL SOURCE
84–01 T84 B140 SW2, pp. 45–75	Croonian lectures on the evolution and dissolution of the nervous system. Delivered at the Royal College of Physicians By-line.	*Lancet*, 1884, **i**: 555–558 29 Mar 84
84–02 T84 SW2, pp. 45–75	The Croonian lectures on evolution and dissolution of the nervous system. Delivered at the Royal College of Physicians, March, 1884 By-line.	*Br Med J*, 1884, **i**: 591–593 29 Mar 84
84–03 T84 B140 SW2, pp. 45–75	Croonian lectures on evolution and dissolution of the nervous system. Delivered at the Royal College of Physicians By-line.	*Med Times Gaz*, 1884, **i**: 411–413 29 Mar 84
84–04 T84 SW2, pp. 45–75	The Croonian lectures on evolution and dissolution of the nervous system. Delivered at the Royal College of Physicians, March, 1884 By-line.	*Br Med J*, 1884, **i**: 660–663 5 Apr 84
84–05 T84 B140 SW2, pp. 45–75	Croonian lectures on evolution and dissolution of the nervous system. Delivered at the Royal College of Physicians By-line.	*Med Times Gaz*, 1884, **i**: 445–448 5 Apr 84
84–06 T84 B140 SW2, pp. 45–75	Croonian lectures on evolution and dissolution of the nervous system. Delivered at the Royal College of Physicians By-line.	*Lancet*, 1884, **i**: 649–652 12 Apr 84
84–07 T84 SW2, pp. 45–75	The Croonian lectures on evolution and dissolution of the nervous system. Delivered at the Royal College of Physicians, March, 1884 By-line.	*Br Med J*, 1884, **i**: 703–707 12 Apr 84

ID	TITLE	PERIODICAL SOURCE
84–08 T84 B140 SW2, pp. 45–75	Croonian lectures on evolution and dissolution of the nervous system. Delivered at the Royal College of Physicians By-line.	*Med Times Gaz*, 1884, **i**: 485–487 18 Apr 84
84–09	The Croonian lectures Report of lectures by HJ	*Med Times Gaz*, 1884, **i**: 529–530 19 Apr 84
84–10 T84 B140 SW2, pp. 45–75	Croonian lectures on evolution and dissolution of the nervous system. Delivered at the Royal College of Physicians By-line.	*Lancet*, 1884, **i**: 739–744 26 Apr 82
84–11 T84 B142	Evolution and dissolution of the nervous system By-line.	*Popular Science Monthly*, 1884, **25**: 171–180 Issue dated Nov 1884
84–12 T84 B141	A case of convulsive seizure beginning in the right foot owing to cortical tumour of the left cerebral hemisphere By-line.	*Proc Med Soc London*, 1882, **6**:151–152 Volume printed 1884

1885

ID	TITLE	PERIODICAL SOURCE
85–01 T85	Royal Medical and Chirurgical Society. The experimental production of chorea and other results of capillary embolism Report of HJ's discussion of a paper read by Dr Angel Money.	*Med Times Gaz*, 1885, **i**: 730–731 30 May 85
85–02	Reviews and notices of books. A treatise on the diseases of the nervous system. By James Ross By-line.	*Brain*, 1885, **8**: 423–425 Issue dated Oct 85
85–03 T85	Medical Society of London. The clinical significance of the deep reflexes Report of HJ's discussion of a paper by Gowers.	*Br Med J*, 1885, **ii**: 867–870 7 Nov 85
85–04 T85 B 144 SW2, pp. 246–250	The Bowman Lecture. Ophthalmology and diseases of the nervous system. Delivered before the Ophthalmological Society, Nov 13th, 1885 By-line.	*Lancet*, 1885, **ii**: 935–938 21 Nov 85
85–05 T85 B143 SW2, pp. 246–250	The Bowman Lecture. Ophthalmology and diseases of the nervous system. Delivered before the Ophthalmological Society, Friday, November 13th By-line.	*Br Med J*, 1885, **ii**: 945–949 21 Nov 85
85–06	The Bowman lecture Report of lecture by HJ.	*Br Med J*, 1885, **ii**: 980–981 21 Nov 85
85–07 T85 B144 SW2, pp. 346–358	Ophthalmology and diseases of the nervous system. Being the Bowman lecture, delivered before the Ophthalmological Society of the United Kingdom, Friday November 13, 1885 By-line.	*Med Times Gaz*, 1885, **ii**: 695–701 21 Nov 85

ID	TITLE	PERIODICAL SOURCE
85–08	The Bowman Lecture	*Med Times Gaz*, 1885, **ii**: 743
	Report of lecture by HJ.	28 Nov 85

1886

ID	TITLE	PERIODICAL SOURCE
86–01 T86 B146	Harveian Society. Paralysis of tongue, palate, and vocal cord Report of case presentation by HJ.	*Lancet*, 1886, i: 689–690 10 Apr 86
86–02 T86 B149 SW1, pp. 348–361	A contribution to the comparative study of convulsions By-line.	*Brain*, 1886, **9**: 1–23 Issue dated Apr 86
86–03	Brain-surgery Report of HJ's discussion of a paper read by Victor Horsley.	*Br Med J*, 1886, ii: 670–675 9 Oct 86
86–04 T86 B148	Medical Society of London. A rare case of epilepsy—Epileptic guinea-pigs Report of case presentation by HJ.	*Lancet*, 1886, ii: 975–976 20 Nov 86
86–05 T86 B147 SW1, pp. 362–365	On a case of fits resembling those artificially produced in guinea-pigs By-line.	*Br Med J*, 1886, ii: 962–963 20 Nov 86
86–06	Harveian Society. Paraplegia in Pott's disease Report of case presentation by HJ.	*Br Med J*, 1886, ii: 977 20 Nov 86
86–07 T85 B145	Ophthalmology and diseases of the nervous system, being the Bowman lecture, delivered Friday, November 13th, 1885 By-line.	*Trans Ophthalmol Soc UK*, 1886, **6**: 1–22 Volume printed 1886

ID	TITLE	PERIODICAL SOURCE
86–08	Graves's disease	*Trans Ophthalmol Soc UK*, 1886, **6**: 58–59
	Report of HJ's discussion at a meeting of the Council of the Ophthalmological Society of the UK.	Volume printed 1886

1887

ID	TITLE	PERIODICAL SOURCE
87–01 T87 B154	Case of left crural monoplegia with subcortical disease: fracture of left femur, which was cancerous By-line.	*Trans Clinical Soc London*, 1887, **20**: 134–136 Volume dated 1887
87–02 T87 B150	Clinical Society of London. Paralysis of the left leg from subcortical disease, with cancer and fracture of the left femur Report of paper read by HJ.	*Br Med J*, 1887, **i**: 510 5 Mar 87
87–03 T87 B151	Medical Society of London. Random association of nervous symptoms with syphilis. Facial monoplegia Report of case presentation by HJ.	*Lancet*, 1887, **i**: 680 2 Apr 87
87–04 T87 B152	Medical Society of London. A case of hemianopsia, and of wasting and paralysis on one side of the tongue in a syphilitic patient Report of case presentation by HJ.	*Br Med J*, 1887, **i**: 729 2 Apr 87
87–05 T87 B156 SW2, pp. 76–91	Remarks on evolution and dissolution of the nervous system By-line.	*J Mental Sci*, 1887, **33**: 25–48 Issue dated Apr 87
87–06	The 'muscular sense'; its nature and cortical localisation Report of HJ's discussion of paper read by H Charlton Bastian at the Neurological Society.	*Brain*, 1887, **10**: 107–109 Issue dated Apr 87

ID	TITLE	PERIODICAL SOURCE
87–07 T87 B159 SW2, pp. 359–364	Remarks on the psychology of joking, delivered at the Medical Society of London, October 17th, 1887 By-line.	*Lancet*, 1887, **ii**: 800–801 22 Oct 87
87–08 B159 SW2, pp. 359–364	An address on the psychology of joking, delivered at the opening of the Medical Society of London, October, 1887 By-line.	*Br Med J*, 1887, **ii**: 870–871 22 Oct 87
87–09	Medical Society of London. Removal of cerebral tumour Report of case presentation by HJ.	*Br Med J*, 1887, **ii**: 997 5 Nov 87
87–10 T87 B153 SW2, pp. 92–118	Remarks on evolution and dissolution of the nervous system By-line.	*Med Press Circular*, 1887, **95**: 461–462 16 Nov 87
87–11 T87 SW2, pp. 92–118	Remarks on evolution and dissolution of the nervous system By-line.	*Med Press Circular*, 1887, **95**: 491–492 23 Nov 87
87–12 T87 SW2, pp. 92–118	Remarks on evolution and dissolution of the nervous system By-line.	*Med Press Circular*, 1887, **95**: 511–513 30 Nov 87
87–13 T87 SW2, pp. 92–118	Remarks on evolution and dissolution of the nervous system By-line.	*Med Press Circular*, 1887, **95**: 586–588 21 Dec 87

ID	TITLE	PERIODICAL SOURCE
87–14 T87 SW2, pp. 92–118	Remarks on evolution and dissolution of the nervous system By-line.	*Med Press Circular*, 1887, **95**: 617–620 28 Dec 87
87–15 T86 SW1, pp. 362–365	On a case of fits resembling those artificially produced in guinea-pigs By-line.	*Proc Med Soc London*, 1886, **10**: 78–85 Volume printed 1887

1888

ID	TITLE	PERIODICAL SOURCE
88–01 T88 SW2, pp. 472–476	Muscular hypertonicity in paralysis Report of HJ's discussion of a paper read by A Hughes Bennett.	*Brain*, 1888, **10**: 312–318 Issue dated Jan 88
88–02 T88	The Medico-Psychological Association Report of discussion by HJ of case presented by Dr Savage.	*J Mental Sci*, 1888, **34**: 145–147 Issue dated Apr 88
88–03 T88 B158 SW2, pp. 365–392	Remarks on the diagnosis and treatment of diseases of the brain By-line.	*Br Med J*, 1888, **ii**: 59–63 14 July 88
88–04 T88 B158 SW2, pp. 365–392	Remarks on the diagnosis and treatment of diseases of the brain By-line.	*Br Med J*, 1888, **ii**: 111–117 21 July 88
88–05 T88 B161 SW1, pp. 385–405	On a particular variety of epilepsy ("intellectual aura"), one case with symptoms of organic brain disease By-line.	*Brain*, 1888, **11**: 179–207 Issue dated July 88
88–06 T88 SW2, pp. 477–481	Inhibition Report of HJ's discussion of a lecture by Dr C Mercier.	*Brain*, 1888, **11**: 386–393 Issue dated Oct 88

ID	TITLE	PERIODICAL SOURCE
88–07 T88 B160 SW1, pp. 366–384	On post-epileptic states: a contribution to the comparative study of insanities By-line.	*J Mental Sci*, 1888, **34**: 349–365 Issue dated Oct 88
88–08 T88 B157	Medical Society of London. Monday, December 27, 1888. Case of paralysis of the lower part of trapezius Report of case presented by HJ.	*Br Med J*, 1888, **ii**: 1393–1394 22 Dec 88
88–09 T87 B159 SW2, pp. 359–364	Opening address By-lined commentary on the neurology of joking.	*Proc Med Soc London*, 1888, **11**: 1–7 Volume printed 1888
88–10 B155	Case in which a cerebral tumour had been removed By-line.	*Proc Med Soc London*, 1888, **11**: 298 Volume printed 1888

1889

ID	TITLE	PERIODICAL SOURCE
89–01 T88 B160 SW1, pp. 366–384	On post-epileptic states: a contribution to the comparative study of insanities By-line.	*J Mental Sci*, 1889, **34**: 490–500 Issue dated Jan 89
89–02 T89 B163	Malposition of the scapula from paralysis of the lower part of the trapezius By-line.	*Illustrated Medical News*, 1889, **2**: 100–101 2 Feb 89
89–03 T89 SW1, pp. 406–411	Medical Society of London. Epilepsy with olfactory aura Report of paper read by HJ and Dr Beevor.	*Lancet*, 1889, **i**: 381 23 Feb 89
89–04 T89 B162 SW2, pp. 393–410	Address in medicine by J. Hughlings Jackson. On the comparative study of diseases of the nervous system By-line.	*Br Med J*, 1889, **ii**: 355–362 17 Aug 89
89–05	Abstract of the address in medicine delivered at the meeting of the British Medical Association, Leeds, by J. Hughlings Jackson. On the comparative study of diseases of the nervous system By-line.	*Lancet*, 1889, **ii**: 355–357 17 Aug 89
89–06	On the comparative study of diseases of the nervous system By-line.	*Med Record*, 1889, **38**: 225–232 31 Aug 89
89–07 T89 B164	Presidential address on ophthalmology and general medicine, delivered before the Ophthalmological Society of the United Kingdom By-line.	*Lancet*, 1889, **ii**: 837–839 26 Oct 89

ID	TITLE	PERIODICAL SOURCE
89–08	Ophthalmological Society. Presidential address Report of lecture delivered by HJ.	*Lancet*, 1889, **ii**: 854–855 26 Oct 89
89–09	Presidential address on ophthalmology and general medicine, delivered before the Ophthalmological Society of the United Kingdom By-line.	*Br Med J*, 1889, **ii**: 911–913 26 Oct 89
89–10 T89 B166 SW1, pp. 406–411	Case of tumour of the right temporo-sphenoidal lobe bearing on the localisation of the sense of smell and on the interpretation of a particular variety of epilepsy By-line HJ and Charles E Beevor.	*Brain*, 1889, **12**: 346–357 Issue dated Oct 89
89–11	Ophthalmological Society of the United Kingdom. Note on a case of hereditary tendency to cataract in early childhood Report of discussion by HJ of paper read by Dr Tatham Thompson.	*Br Med J*, 1889, **ii**: 1835 31 Dec 89
89–12 T89 B165	Paralysis of trapezius Report of case presented by HJ.	*Proc Med Soc London*, 1888, **12**: 285–286 Volume printed 1889

1890

ID	TITLE	PERIODICAL SOURCE
90–01	On rigidity with exaggerated tendon reactions, and cerebellar influx By-lined letter.	*Br Med J*, 1890, **i**: 541 8 Mar 90
90–02 T90 B167 SW1, pp. 412–357	The Lumleian Lectures on convulsive seizures By-line.	*Lancet*, 1890, **i**: 685–688 29 Mar 90
90–03 T90 SW1, pp. 412–357	The Lumleian Lectures on convulsive seizures, delivered before the Royal College of Physicians of London By-line.	*Br Med J*, 1890, **i**: 703–707 29 Mar 90
90–04 T90 B167 SW1, pp. 412–357	The Lumleian Lectures on convulsive seizures By-line.	*Lancet*, 1890, **i**: 735–738 5 Apr 90
90–05 T90 SW1, pp. 412–357	The Lumleian Lectures on convulsive seizures, delivered before the Royal College of Physicians of London By-line.	*Br Med J*, 1890, **i**: 765–771 5 Apr 90
90–06 T90 B167 SW1, pp. 412–357	The Lumleian Lectures on convulsive seizures By-line.	*Lancet*, 1890, **i**: 785–788 12 Apr 90
90–07 T90 SW1, pp. 412–357	The Lumleian Lectures on convulsive seizures, delivered before the Royal College of Physicians of London By-line.	*Br Med J*, 1890, **i**: 821–827 12 Apr 90

ID	TITLE	PERIODICAL SOURCE
90–08 T89 B164	Presidential address, delivered at the first meeting of the session, October 17th, 1889 No by-line, but identical to 89–08, which carries by-line.	*Trans Ophthalmol Soc UK*, 1890, **10**: xliv–lix Volume printed 1890

1891

ID	TITLE	PERIODICAL SOURCE
91–01 T91	Medical Society of London. Treadler's cramp	*Lancet*, 1891, **i**: 434
	Report of case presented by W H R Rivers for HJ.	21 Feb 91
91–02	Hunterian Society. Phonographic illustration of disease	*Br Med J*, 1891, **i**: 644–645
	Report of presentation of phonographic recording of abnormal speech by HJ and W H R Rivers.	21 Mar 91
91–03	Hunterian Society. Phonographic illustration of disease	*Lancet*, 1891, **i**: 884
	Report of presentation of phonographic recording of abnormal speech by HJ and Dr Rivers.	18 Apr 91
91–04	Clinical Society of London. Pseudo-hypertrophic paralysis	*Lancet*, 1891, **i**: 988
	Report of case presented by Dr J Taylor for HJ.	2 May 91
91–05 T91 B168	Remarks on a case of return of knee-jerks after hemiplegia in a tabetic	*Br Med J*, 1891, **ii**: 57–58
	By-line HJ and James Taylor.	11 July 91
91–06 T91	A case of treadler's cramp	*Brain*, 1891, **14**: 110–111
	By-line W H R Rivers of case under the care of HJ.	Volume printed 1891

1892

ID	TITLE	PERIODICAL SOURCE
92–01 T92 B171	Note on the knee-jerk in the condition of super-venosity By-line.	*Br Med J*, 1892, **i**: 326 13 Feb 92
92–02 T92 B172	A case of syringomyelus By-line HJ and James Galloway.	*Lancet*, 1892, **i**: 408–411 20 Feb 92
92–03 T92 B173	Lecture on neurological fragments. Delivered before the Hunterian Society By-line.	*Br Med J*, 1892, **i**: 487–492 5 Mar 92
92–04 T92 B173	Lecture on neurological fragments. Delivered before the Hunterian Society By-line.	*Lancet*, 1892, **i**: 511–514 5 Mar 92
92–05 T92 B174	A case of double hemiplegia with bulbar symptoms By-line HJ and James Taylor.	*Lancet*, 1892, **ii**: 1320–1322 10 Dec 92
92–06 T92 B170	Case of Friedreich's ataxy By-line.	*Trans Med Soc London*, 1892, **15**: 462 Volume printed 1892

1893

ID	TITLE	PERIODICAL SOURCE
93–01 T93 B175	Neurological fragments. No. I. Two cases of ophthalmoplegia externa with paresis of the orbicularis palpebrarum (Illustration of Mendel's hypothesis) By-line.	*Lancet*, 1893, **ii**: 128–129 15 July 93
93–02 T93 B176 SW2, pp. 205–212	Words and other symbols in mentation By-line.	*Med Press Circular*, 1893, **107**: 205–208 30 Aug 93

1894

ID	TITLE	PERIODICAL SOURCE
94–01 T94 B177	Neurological fragments. No. II. Congenital ptosis—innervation of the upper eyelid By-line.	*Lancet*, 1894, i: 11 6 Jan 94
94–02 T94	Neurological fragments. No. III. On the use of cocaine in the investigation of certain abnormal motorial conditions of the eyes By-line.	*Lancet*, 1894, i: 11–12 6 Jan 94
94–03 T94 B178	Neurological fragments. No. IV. On the pupil and eyelids in cases of paralysis of the cervical sympathetic nerve By-line.	*Lancet*, 1894, i: 12 6 Jan 94
94–04 T94 B179	Neurological fragments. No. V. Dr. Risien Russell's researches on the knee-jerks during artificially induced asphyxia in dogs and rabbits By-line.	*Lancet*, 1894, i: 134–135 20 Jan 94
94–05 T94	Neurological fragments. No. VI. The knee-jerks in two cases of opium poisoning By-line.	*Lancet*, 1894, i: 135 20 Jan 94
94–06 T94 B180	Neurological fragments. No. VII. Temporo-sphenoidal (left) abscess from ear disease; right hemiplegia, with lateral deviation of the eyes and aphasia; trephining; recovery By-line.	*Lancet*, 1894, i: 390–392 17 Feb 94
94–07 T94 B181	A clinical study of a case of cyst of the cerebellum: weakness of spinal muscles: death from failure of respiration By-line HJ and J S Risien Russell.	*Br Med J*, 1894, i: 393–395 24 Feb 94

ID	TITLE	PERIODICAL SOURCE
94–08 T94 B182	Neurological fragments. No. VIII. Intensification of lateral deviation of the eyes in a case of hemiplegia during chloroform anaesthesia; Dr. Risien Russell's researches on reappearance under anaesthesia of lateral deviation of the eyes in dogs recovered from that deviation which had been produced by ablation of part of the eye area of the cerebral cortex, and on lateral deviation of the eyes in intact dogs when under ether By-line.	*Lancet*, 1894, **i**: 1052–1053 28 Apr 94
94–09 T94	Neurological fragments. No. IX. Further remarks on lateral deviation of the eyes; Dr. Risien Russell's researches on representation of various ocular movements in the cerebral cortex; slight degrees of lateral deviation of the eyes; "punctuation" of motion of the eyeballs (trivial nystagmus) in some cases of hemiplegia By-line.	*Lancet*, 1894, **i**: 1053–1054 28 Apr 94
94–10 T94 B187 SW2, pp. 411–421	The factors of insanities By-line.	*Med Press Circular*, 1894, **108**: 615–619 13 June 94
94–11 T94 B183	A further note on the return of the knee-jerk in a tabetic patient after an attack of hemiplegia By-line HJ and James Taylor.	*Br Med J*, 1894, **i**: 1350–1351 23 June 94
94–12 T94 B184	Neurological fragments. No. X. On slight and severe cerebral paroxysms (epileptic attacks) with auditory warning; slight paroxysms with deafness and the special imperception called "word-blindness"; spectral words (auditory); inability to speak and to write By-line.	*Lancet*, 1894, **ii**: 182–183 28 July 94

ID	TITLE	PERIODICAL SOURCE
94–13 T94 B185	Neurological fragments. No. XI. Cerebral paroxysms (epileptic attacks) with an auditory warning; in slight seizures the special imperceptions called "word-deafness" (Wernicke) and "word-blindness" (Kussmaul); inability to speak and spectral words (auditory and visual) By-line.	*Lancet*, 1894, **ii**: 252–253 8 Aug 94
94–14	Testimonial to Dr. Hughlings Jackson Report of preparation for retirement testimonial to HJ.	*Lancet*, 1894, **ii**: 1362 8 Dec 94
94–15 T94 B186	Neurological fragments. No. XII. Absent knee-jerks in some cases of pneumonia. Inaction of the intercostal muscles in respiration with good voluntary action of the same muscles, in a case of "latent pneumonia" By-line.	*Lancet*, 1894, **ii**: 1472–1473 22 Dec 94

1895

ID	TITLE	PERIODICAL SOURCE
95–01 T95 B188	Neurological fragments. No. XIII. Fits following touching the head—A case published by Dr. Dunsmure (1874) By-line.	*Lancet*, 1895, **i**: 274–275 2 Feb 95
95–02 T95 B189	Neurological fragments. No. XIV. The lowest level of central nervous system—the study of tabes dorsalis and some other nervous maladies, as owing to disease of this level and its immediate connexions. By-line.	*Lancet*, 1895, **i**: 394–396 16 Feb 95
95–03 T95 B190	Neurological fragments. No. XV. Superior and subordinate centres of the lowest level By-line.	*Lancet*, 1895, **i**: 476–478 23 Feb 95
95–04	London Hospital. Presentation of testimonial to Dr. Hughlings Jackson, F.R.S., by Sir James Paget Report of testimonial to HJ.	*Br Med J*, 1895, **ii**: 861–863 5 Oct 95
95–05	Presentation to Dr. Hughlings Jackson Report of testimonial to HJ.	*Lancet*, 1895, **ii**: 857 5 Oct 95
95–06	The testimonial to Dr. Hughlings Jackson, F.R.S. Report of testimonial to HJ.	*London Hospital Gazette*, 1895, **2**: 34–39 Issue dated Oct 95

ID	TITLE	PERIODICAL SOURCE
95–07 T95 SW2, pp. 482–484	On imperative ideas. Being a discussion of Dr. Hack Tuke's paper (*Brain*, 1894) 1—Dr. Hughlings-Jackson By-line.	*Brain*, 1895, **18**: 318–322 Volume dated 1895

1896

ID	TITLE	PERIODICAL SOURCE
96–01 T96 B191	Neurological fragments. No. XVI. The lowest level—Negative and positive symptoms—The physiological element in symptomatologies—Remarks on the symptomatology of fracture-dislocations of the spine crushing the cervical cord completely across below the emergence of the phrenic nerves—Charlton Bastian's researches on complete transverse lesions of the cord above the cervical enlargement; loss of the knee-jerks from these lesions; observations by Sherrington By-line.	*Lancet*, 1896, **ii**: 1662–1664 12 Dec 96

1897

ID	TITLE	PERIODICAL SOURCE
97–01 T97 B192	Neurological fragments. No. XVII. Cervical fracture-dislocation cases—Destruction by complete transverse lesion of the cervical cord of intrinsic and extrinsic elements of the lowest level—Paralysis "at" and paralysis "below" the lesion—Mutilation of the nervous mechanisms of the "four systems" (thermal, circulatory, respiratory, digestive)—Intra-central inhibition By-line.	*Lancet*, 1897, **i**: 18–23 2 Jan 97

1898

ID	TITLE	PERIODICAL SOURCE
98–01 T98 B193 SW2, pp. 422–443	The Hughlings Jackson lecture on the relations of different divisions of the central nervous system to one another and to parts of the body. Delivered before the Neurological Society, Dec. 8th, 1897 By-line.	*Lancet*, 1898, **i**: 79–87 8 Jan 98
98–02 T98 B193 SW2, pp. 422–443	Remarks on the relations of different divisions of the central nervous system to one another and to parts of the body. Delivered before the Neurological Society, December 8th, 1897 By-line.	*Br Med J*, 1898, **i**: 65–69 8 Jan 98
98–03 T98 SW1, pp. 458–463	Case of epilepsy with tasting movements and "dreamy state"—very small patch of softening in the left uncinate gyrus By-line HJ and Walter S Colman.	*Brain*, 1898, **21**: 580–590 Volume printed 1898

1899

ID	TITLE	PERIODICAL SOURCE
99–01 T99 B194 B195	Neurological fragments. No. XVIII. On asphyxia in slight epileptic paroxysms—On the symptomatology of slight epileptic fits supposed to depend on discharge-lesions of the uncinate gyrus By-line.	*Lancet*, 1899, **i**: 79–80 14 Jan 99
99–02 T99 B196	Neurological fragments. No. XIX. A case of left hemiplegia with turning of the eyes to the right—slightly greater amplitude of movement of the left side of the chest in inspiration proper: and slightly less amplitude of movement of that side in voluntary expansion of the chest By-line.	*Lancet*, 1899, **ii**: 1659–1660 16 Dec 99
99–03 T99 SW2, pp. 464–473	Epileptic attacks with a warning of a crude sensation of smell and with the intellectual aura (dreamy state) in a patient who had symptoms pointing to gross organic disease of the right temporo-sphenoidal lobe By-line HJ and Purves Stewart.	*Brain*, 1899, **22**: 534–549 Volume printed 1899
99–04 T99 SW2, pp. 444–451	Remarks on loss of movements of the intercostal muscles in some cases of surgical anaesthesia by chloroform and ether By-line HJ and James S Collier.	*Brain*, 1899, **22**: 550–562 Volume printed 1899
99–05 T99 SW2, pp. 452–458	On certain relations of the cerebrum and cerebellum (on rigidity of hemiplegia and on paralysis agitans) By-line.	*Brain*, 1899, **22**: 621–630 Volume printed 1899

1900

ID	TITLE	PERIODICAL SOURCE
00–01	Epileptic attacks with crude sensations of smell and an intellectual aura Report of paper by HJ and Purves Stewart.	*Lancet*, 1900, **i**: 477 17 Feb 1900
00–02	The medical staff and the management of the National Hospital for the Paralysed and Epileptic, Queen Square By-lined letter by HJ, *et al.*	*Lancet*, 1900, **ii**: 351–352 4 Aug 1900

1901

ID	TITLE	PERIODICAL SOURCE
01–01	Sprengel's shoulder	*Polyclinic*, 1901, **3**: 102–104
	Report of HJ case presentation, with reprint of *Illustrated Medical News*, 1889, **2**: 100–101.	Issue dated Oct 01

1902

ID	TITLE	PERIODICAL SOURCE
02–01 T02 B197	Neurological fragments. No. XX. Lowest level fits —Hypothesis on the mechanism of laryngeal crisis in tabes dorsalis—The physiological factor in symptomatologies—Remarks on some other lowest level fits—Terminal tonic spasms By-line.	*Lancet*, 1902, **i**: 727–731 15 Mar 02
02–02 T02 SW1, pp. 474–481	Observations on a case of convulsions (trunk fit or lowest level fit?) By-line HJ and H Douglas Singer.	*Brain*, 1902, **25**: 122–132 Volume printed 1902
02–03 T02 SW1, pp. 482–486	Further observations on a case of convulsions (trunk fit or lowest level fit?) By-line HJ and Stanley Barnes.	*Brain* 1902, **25**: 286–292 Note pagination error in original. Volume printed 1902

1903

ID	TITLE	PERIODICAL SOURCE
03–01	On the study of diseases of the nervous system. A lecture delivered June, 1864. Reprinted from the *London Hospital Reports*, vol. i, 1864, at the special request of Sir William Broadbent By-line.	*Brain*, 1903, **26**: 367–382 Volume dated 1903
03–02	On aural vertigo By–line.	*Polyclinic*, 1903, **5**: 98–101 Volume dated 1903

1906

ID	TITLE	PERIODICAL SOURCE
06–01 T06	Case of tumour of middle lobe of cerebellum—cerebellar paralysis with rigidity (cerebellar attitude)—occasional tetanus-like seizures (1871) By-line.	*Brain*, 1906, **29**: 425–440 Volume printed 1907
06–02 T06	Case of tumour of middle lobe of cerebellum. Cerebellar attitude. No tetanus-like seizures. General remarks on the cerebellar attitude (1872) By-line.	*Brain*, 1906, **29**: 441–445 Volume printed 1907

1907

ID	TITLE	PERIODICAL SOURCE
07–01 T07	Obituary. Sir William Broadbent	*Br Med J*, 1907, **ii**: 180–181
	By-lined letter.	20 July 07
07–02 T07	Announcement	*Lancet*, 1907, **ii**: 1632–1633
	Report of placement of bust of HJ in the hall of the National Hospital, Queen Square.	7 Dec 07
07–03	Announcement	*Br Med J*, 1907, **ii**: 1738
	Report of placement of bust of HJ in the hall of the National Hospital, Queen Square.	14 Dec 07

1909

ID	TITLE	PERIODICAL SOURCE
09–01 T09	Neurological fragments. No. XXI. Remarks on certain abnormalities of the sensations heat and cold—Illustration of physiological antagonism By-line.	*Lancet*, 1909, i: 377–378 6 Feb 09
09–02 T09 SW2, pp. 459–471	On some abnormalities of ocular movements, with particular reference to "erroneous projection" in cases of paralysis of muscles of the eye-ball, especially in cases of paralysis of an external rectus—out-going (centro-peripheral) *v.* in-going (periphero-central) currents By-line HJ and Leslie Paton.	*Lancet* 1909, i: 900–904 27 Mar 09

Appendix 1

Pamphlets of John Hughlings Jackson, Rockefeller Medical Library, Institute of Neurology, University College London

The archives of the Rockefeller Medical Library hold a collection of pamphlets written by John Hughlings Jackson, the only such collection known to exist. Most of these pamphlets reprint articles published in contemporaneous medical periodicals, though one pamphlet was not published elsewhere. There is internal evidence that Hughlings Jackson circulated these pamphlets privately. Some contain marginal comments and corrections in Hughlings Jackson's hand, and in other hands as well.

The Rockefeller Medical Library collection contains five boxes of loose items, which are labelled boxes A–E. Each item is assigned a serial number in the order in which it appears in the collection. The identification number consists of the box letter followed by the serial number.

A3. Suggestions for studying diseases of the nervous system on Professor Owen's vertebral theory
50-page pamphlet. London, H K Lewis, 1863. Preface dated 5 January 1863, at 5 Queen Square. No marginalia. Included in Taylor's and Greenblatt's bibliographies.

A11. On a case of muscular atrophy, with disease of the spinal cord and medulla oblongata
8-page pamphlet. London, J E Adlard, 1867. Authors: J Lockhart Clarke, J Hughlings Jackson. Reprinted from *Trans Medico-Chirurgical Soc*, series 2, 1867, **32**: 489–499. No marginalia.

A15. Cases of disease of the nervous system in patients the subject of inherited syphilis
22-page pamphlet. London, John Churchill and Sons, 1868. Reprinted with alterations from *Transactions of the St Andrews Medical Graduates Association, 1867*, 1868, **1**: 146–160. Two copies, one with inscription "Written 23 years ago. JHJ" in red ink, and other marginal comments in Hughlings Jackson's hand.

A16. Notes on the physiology and pathology of the nervous system
8-page pamphlet. London, B Pardon and Sons, undated. Reprinted from *Med Times Gaz*, 1868, **ii**: 526–528. No marginalia.

A18. Observations on the physiology and pathology of hemi-chorea
12-page pamphlet Edinburgh, Oliver and Boyd, 1868. Reprinted from *Edinburgh Med J*, 1868, **14**, 294–303. Bottom of pages 11–12 cut off. No marginalia.

Appendix 1

A19. Observations on defects of sight in brain disease, and ophthalmoscopic examination during sleep
15-page pamphlet. London, Harrison and Sons, 1863. Reprinted from *Royal London Ophthalmic Hospital Reports*, 1863, **4**: 10–19 and 35–37.

A25. A study of convulsions
45-page pamphlet. London, Odell & Ives, 1870. Reprinted from *Transactions of the St Andrews Medical Graduates Association, 1869*, 1870, **3**: 162–204. Two copies. Copy no. 1 has marginal notes in unknown hand. Copy no. 2 is signed PW (illegible).

A29. On the anatomical, physiological, and pathological investigations of epilepsies
36-page pamphlet. London, Spottiswood and Co., undated. Reprinted from *West Riding Lunatic Asylum Medical Reports*, 1873, **3**: 315–349. Two copies. Copy no. 1 carries printed cover "From the author", with written inscription. Copy no. 2 contains editing marks and notes in pencil and pen.

A30. Clinical and physiological researches on the nervous system. No. 1. On the localisation of movements in the brain
25-page pamphlet plus xlvii page preface, London, J and A Churchill, 1875. Reprinted from a series from *Lancet*, 1873. Marginal editing notes, comments and corrections.

A33. Observations on the localisation of movements in the cerebral hemispheres, as revealed by cases of convulsion, chorea and "aphasia"
23-page pamphlet. London, Spottiswood & Co., undated. Reprinted from *West Riding Lunatic Asylum Medical Reports*, 1873, **3**: 175–195. Title-page inscribed in Hughlings Jackson's hand.

A34. A physician's notes on ophthalmology
37-page pamphlet. London, Harrison and Sons, undated. Title-page contains the note: "Chiefly reprinted, with alterations, from the Royal London Ophthalmic Hospital Reports, vol. VII, part 4, 1873, and vol. VIII, part 1, 1874". No marginalia. Mentioned in Taylor's bibliography.

A43. A physician's notes on ophthalmology
37-page pamphlet. London, Harrison and Sons, undated. Title-page carries note: "Reprinted from the Periscope of the Royal London Ophthalmic Hospital Reports Vol VIII, part 2, 1875." No marginalia.

A44. Nervous symptoms in cases of congenital syphilis
Pamphlet. Lewes, Geo. P. Bacon, undated. Carries note: "Reprinted from Journal of Mental Science, January, 1875." No marginalia.

Appendix 1

A46. The syphilitic affections of the nervous system
19-page pamphlet. Lewes, Geo. P. Bacon, undated. Title-page carries note: "Reprinted from Journal of Mental Science, Jul, 1875." No marginalia.

A48. On ocular movements, with vertigo, produced by pressure on a diseased ear
5-page pamphlet. London, Adlard, undated. Reprinted from *Trans Ophthalmol Soc UK*, 1883, **3**: 261–265. Two copies, copy no. 1 with editing marks.

A49. A case of double optic neuritis without cerebral tumour
13-page pamphlet. London, Harrison and Sons, undated. Reprinted from *Royal London Ophthalmic Hospital Reports*, 1876, **8**: 445–455. Issue dated May 1876. Three copies. Copy no. 1 stamped "E. Arnold Carmichael" and inscribed "J. Hughlings Jackson" in an unknown hand. No marginalia.

A50. Case of large cerebral tumour without optic neuritis and with left hemiplegia and imperception
Pamphlet. London, Harrison and Sons, undated. Reprinted from *Royal London Ophthalmic Hospital Reports*, 1876, **8**: 434–444. Issue dated May 1876. Two copies. Copy no. 1 inscribed "From the Royal London Ophthalmic Hospital Reports May 1876 (Vol 8 Part 3)", with marginal comments in Hughlings Jackson's hand. Copy no. 2 stamped "E. Arnold Carmichael".

A52. On nervous symptoms with ear disease
10-page pamphlet. London, publisher not given, dated 1877. Reprinted from *Br Med J*, 1877, **i**: 349–351. Three copies. Marginal corrections in Hughlings Jackson's hand.

A55. Remarks on the routine use of the ophthalmoscope in cerebral disease
23-page pamphlet. London, Steam Printing Works, 1879. Reprinted from *Med Press Circular*, 1879, **27**: 439–441, 459–461, 479–480. No marginalia. Mentioned in Taylor's bibliography.

A57. On eye symptoms in locomotor ataxy
16-page pamphlet. London, J E Adlard, undated. Reprinted from *Trans Ophthalmol Soc UK*, 1881, **1**: 139–154. Two copies. No marginalia.

A59. Discussion on the relation between optic neuritis and intracranial disease
35-page pamphlet. London, J E Adlard, undated. Reprinted from *Trans Ophthalmol Soc UK*, 1881, **1**: 60–115. Two copies. No marginalia.

A64. The Croonian lectures on evolution and dissolution of the nervous system. Delivered at the Royal College of Physicians, March, 1884
32-page pamphlet. London, British Medical Association, undated. Reprinted from *Br Med J*, 1884, **i**: 591–593, 660–663, 703–707. Two copies. Marginal editing comments.

Appendix 1

A65. Remarks on evolution and dissolution of the nervous system
24-page pamphlet. Lewes, H Wolff, undated. Reprinted from *J Mental Sci*, 1887, **33**: 25–48. Three copies. Copies nos. 1 and 2 contain editing comments. Copy no. 3 is stamped "E. Arnold Carmichael".

A67. On a case of fits resembling those artificially produced in guinea-pigs
8-page pamphlet. London, Harrison and Sons, undated. Reprinted from *Proc Med Soc London*, 1886 [published 1887], **10**: 78–85. Two copies. No marginalia.

A68. Case of left crural monoplegia with subcortical disease: fracture of left femur, which was cancerous
3-page pamphlet. London, Adlard and Son, undated. Reprinted from *Trans Clinical Soc London*, 1887, **20**: 134–136. Four copies. No marginalia.

A69. An address on the psychology of joking, delivered at the opening of the Medical Society of London, October, 1887
4-page pamphlet. London, British Medical Association, undated. Reprinted from *Br Med J*, 1887, **ii**: 870–871. Two copies. Copy no. 1 contains marginal comments in Hughlings Jackson's hand. Copy no. 2 contains a citation in Hughlings Jackson's hand and editing marks in another hand. Copy no. 2 appends a typescript of additional material added to the *Selected Writings*.

A70. Remarks on evolution and dissolution of the nervous system
40-page pamphlet. London, John Bale and Sons, 1888. Three copies. Copy no. 1 contains reference and marginal comments in Hughlings Jackson's hand. Copy no. 2 contains editing notes. Mentioned in Taylor's bibliography.

A71. On post-epileptic states: a contribution to the comparative study of insanities. First instalment
17-page pamphlet. Lewes, H Wolff, undated. Reprinted from *J Mental Sci*, 1888, **34**: 349–365. No marginalia.

A72. On post-epileptic states: a contribution to the comparative study of insanities. Second instalment
10-page pamphlet. Lewes, H Wolff, undated. Reprinted from *J Mental Sci*, 1889, **34**: 490–500. No marginalia. Stamped "E. Arnold Carmichael".

A73. On a particular variety of epilepsy ("intellectual aura"), one case with symptoms of organic brain disease
28-page pamphlet. London, Macmillan and Co., 1888. Reprinted from *Brain*, 1888, **11**: 179–207. No marginalia.

A74. Remarks on the diagnosis and treatment of diseases of the brain
Pamphlet. London, British Medical Association, undated. Rprinted from *Br Med J*, 1888, **ii**: 59–63, 111–117. Three copies. Copy no. 1 inscribed "With best regards.

Appendix 1

JHJ", in Hughlings Jackson's hand. Also note on the title-page: "corrected Oct 30th, 1890". Marginal corrections in Hughlings Jackson's hand. Copy no. 2 contains a reference and corrections in Hughlings Jackson's hand and editing marks in another hand. Copy no. 3 has no marginalia.

A79. The Lumleian Lectures on convulsive seizures, delivered before the Royal College of Physicians of London
47-page pamphlet. London, British Medical Association, undated. Reprinted from *Br Med J*, 1890, **i**: 703–707, 765–771, 821–827. No marginalia.

A84. The factors of insanities
25-page pamphlet. London, Danks & Son, 1894. Reprinted from *Med Press Circular*, 1894, **108**: 615–619. Two copies. No marginalia.

A85. A clinical study of a case of cyst of the cerebellum: Weakness of spinal muscles: Death from failure of respiration
6-page pamphlet. London, British Medical Association, 1894. Authors: J Hughlings Jackson and J S Risien Russell. Reprinted from *Br Med J*, 1894, **i**: 393–395. No marginalia.

A87. On imperative ideas. Being a discussion of Dr. Hack Tuke's paper (*Brain*, 1894). 1— Dr. Hughlings-Jackson
5-page pamphlet. London, Macmillan and Co., 1895. Reprinted from *Brain*, 1895, **18**: 318–322. Editorial comments in unknown hand.

A90. Case of epilepsy with tasting movements and "dreamy state"—very small patch of softening in the left uncinate gyrus
19-page pamphlet. London, Macmillan and Co., 1898. Authors: J Hughlings Jackson and Walter S Colman. Reprinted from *Brain*, 1898, **21**: 580–590. Two copies. No marginalia.

A91. Remarks on loss of movements of the intercostal muscles in some cases of surgical anaesthesia by chloroform and ether
12-page pamphlet. London, Macmillan and Co., 1899. Reprinted from *Brain*, 1899, **22**: 550–562. Authors: J Hughlings Jackson and James S Collier. No marginalia.

A92. On certain relations of the cerebrum and cerebellum (on rigidity of hemiplegia and on paralysis agitans)
9-page pamphlet. London, Macmillan and Co., 1899. Reprinted from *Brain*, 1899, **22**: 621–630. Two copies. Copy no. 1 contains citation and editing marks in unknown hand. Copy no. 2 no marginalia.

A94. Observations on a case of convulsions (trunk fit or lowest level fit?)
10-page pamphlet. London, Macmillan and Co., 1902. Authors: J Hughlings

Appendix 1

Jackson and H Douglas Singer. Reprinted from *Brain*, 1902, **25**: 122–132. Two copies. No marginalia.

A95. Further observations on a case of convulsions (trunk fit or lowest level fit?)
6-page pamphlet. London, Macmillan and Co., 1902. Reprinted from *Brain*, 1902, **25**: 286–292. Authors: J Hughlings Jackson and Stanley Barnes. No marginalia.

A97. Case of tumour of the middle lobe of the cerebellum—cerebellar paralysis with rigidity (cerebellar attitude)—occasional tetanus-like seizures
20-page pamphlet. London, Macmillan and Co., 1906. Reprinted from *Brain*, 1906, **29**: 425–440. Two copies. Copy no. 1 inscribed "to be returned to Dr. James Taylor" and stamped "E. Arnold Carmichael". Copy no. 2 has no marginalia.

Appendix 2

Unpublished Writings of John Hughlings Jackson, Rockefeller Medical Library, Institute of Neurology, University College London

The archives of the Rockefeller Medical Library hold a number of unpublished manuscripts of John Hughlings Jackson, the only ones of his known to exist. These manuscripts are mainly typescripts prepared between 1898 and 1910 in collaboration with James Taylor, but two are handwritten. They are in various stages of completion; most contain marginal comments and corrections in Hughlings Jackson's hand. This catalogue includes forty-five items.

A20. Observations on the physiology of language
    Galley proofs of 41-page pamphlet. London, Wyman and Sons, 1868. Poor repair. One part excised. Some pages cut. No marginalia.

B2. A suggestion for the treatment of epilepsy
    Unpublished typescript. Signed "J. Hughlings Jackson", dated December 5, 1899. Labelled "For private circulation". Marginal note in Hughlings Jackson's hand "(DL means Discharge Lesion)".

B5. On certain supposed ponto-bulbo-spinal (lowest level) fits
    Unpublished typescript. Dated 20/1/1900. Commentary on a case discussed in *Trans Ophthalmol Soc UK,* 1887, **8**: 276. Marginal comment in Hughlings Jackson's hand.

B25. The psychology of joking
    Unpublished typescript. Comments related to 'Remarks on the psychology of joking, delivered at the Medical Society of London, October 17th, 1887', *Lancet,* 1887, **ii**: 800–801.

C20. Out-going or in-going current?
    Typescript. Printed for private circulation. Labelled "Not to be returned." Dated June 6, 1904.

C21. Letter regarding Sir William Gairdner's case
    Unpublished letter, dated November 7, 1903.

C22. Lowest level of the cerebral subsystem
    Unpublished typescript with corrections in Hughlings Jackson's hand. Undated.

Appendix 2

C23. Remarks on ether and chloroform anaesthesia
Unpublished typescript. Labelled "for private circulation." Dated November 20, 1899.

C24. Remarks of the analysis of symptomatologies of paroxysms of epileptic (cerebral) fits
Unpublished typescript with Hughlings Jackson's handwritten corrections. Undated. Pages 7–12 missing.

C25. A case of epileptiform convulsions of the face
Unpublished typescript. Undated. The patient was in the London Hospital, December 1874 to January 1875. Hughlings Jackson is styled F.R.S., so it must have been written after 1878.

C26. Hypothesis on the mechanism of laryngeal crises in tabes dorsalis
Unpublished typescript. Undated; as it refers to 'Neurological Fragments' 1892, clearly written after that.

C27. The analysis of whooping cough
Unpublished manuscript, torn from notebook. Undated. Corrected in red ink.

C28. Remarks on the hierarchy of the nervous system
Unpublished typescript. Undated; refers to a letter from Risien Russell dated November 24, 1898, so written after that. Illegible handwritten note on first page. Some pages cut. Pages 7–12 torn away, left upper corner fragment remains. Includes Sections 1, 2, 5, 6; sections 3 and 4 missing. Last sentence on page 33 incomplete.

C29. Section 4. Risien Russell's researches on the prae-frontal lobe
Unpublished typescript. Undated; refers to the *Lancet* of January 1898, so written after that. Labelled Section 4, could be a re-written section from item C28.

C30. On normal nervous discharges
Unpublished typescript. Undated; refers to a paper published in 1898, so written after that. Handwritten corrections in pencil.

C31. Fits of several kinds—Some with dreamy state, gustatory movements and epigastric sensation (and suffocative feeling?) Fear, eructation. Possibly recession of objects
Unpublished typescript. Undated; refers to a paper published in 1880. Illegible notation. Letter from Weir Mitchell. 2 copies.

C32. Pachymeningitis v. syringomyelia v. tumour
Unpublished typescript. Undated. The patient was seen in January 1893. Handwritten corrections in Hughlings Jackson's hand.

Appendix 2

C33. Vertical vertigo
Unpublished typescript. Undated; mentions a paper published in 1894. Title in Hughlings Jackson's hand, also initialed "JHJ". Handwritten comments and corrections.

C34. On the symptomatology, diagnosis and treatment of syphilitic affections of the brain
Unpublished typescript. Undated; mentions paper of 1873. Marginal comments and corrections in Hughlings Jackson's hand.

C35. Untitled collection of comments on ophthalmology
Typescript of extracts from published papers, with unpublished commentary. Some with corrections.

C36. Untitled analysis of a patient with attacks of unconciousness, or aphasia, or affection of the right arm and leg. First-person account of attacks of aphasia.
Unpublished typescript. The analysis is signed "J. Hughlings Jackson"; the first person account is unsigned. Undated. The two papers are pinned together.

C37. Untitled fragment on treatment of syphilis, pages 27–32.
Unpublished typescript. Unsigned, undated, contains a reference to a paper of 1875. No marginalia or corrections.

C38. Loose paper inscribed "To be kept", in Hughlings Jackson's hand.
Contains 5 items:
A. Offprint of L Pierce Clark, 'The movement of superior intercostal muscles in hemiplegics', *Amer J Medical Sci,* December 1903. Inscribed "To be returned to Dr. JHJ", crossed out, re-inscribed "Dr. Taylor, from JHJ."
B. Tearsheet of Judson S Bury, 'Note on the respiratory movements in hemiplegia', *Lancet,* 19 Dec 1903, **ii**: 1714.
C. Outline on hemiplegia, in Hughlings Jackson's hand.
D. Unpublished note on respiration in hemiplegia, inscribed "Not published. JHJ", dated September 24, 1903.
E. Commentary on respiration beginning "Dr. Hughlings Jackson writes as follows..."

E3. Resistances
Handwritten 26-page notebook bound in red paper. Illegible writing on cover in Hughlings Jackson's hand. Written in the first person singular, but the handwriting is neither Hughlings Jackson's nor Taylor's. Strong suggestion of dictated writing. Material cut from some pages.

E7. Untitled fragment of typescript on epilepsy
Unpublished 78-page typescript, first 5 pages torn away. No title, reference or date. Corrections in Hughlings Jackson's hand. Some pages cut.

Appendix 2

E9. Remarks on the symptomatology of acute and chronic brain disease
Unpublished typescript, corrections in Hughlings Jackson's hand.

E10. Crude sensations and dreamy states (intellectual aurae) as symptoms in certain paroxysms (epileptic fits)
Unpublished typescript, corrections in Hughlings Jackson's hand, unfinished, 4 pages.

E11. Remarks on evolution and dissolution in nervous maladies (with special reference to double mental conditions in paroxysms of uncinate epilepsies and to so-called "procursive epilepsy")—A scheme of levels of the cerebral sub-system—On duality of mentation and of the associated cerebration. (Wigan's subject)
Unpublished typescript, undated, corrections in Hughlings Jackson's hand.

E12. Erroneous projection
Unpublished typescript, undated, corrections in Hughlings Jackson's hand.

E13. The ataxic gait of tabetics
Unpublished typescript, undated; refers to a paper of 1875. Corrections in Hughlings Jackson's hand.

E14. Remarks on the duality of the process of cerebration and of the associated process of mentation ("Wigan's process")
Unpublished typescript, undated, corrections in Hughlings Jackson's hand. Title-page only.

E15. Untitled fragment on localization and psychology.
9-page unpublished typescript, title-page missing, undated. Corrections in Hughlings Jackson's hand.

E16. Untitled commentary on Pierce Clark and epilepsy
5-page unpublished typescript, undated, corrections in Hughlings Jackson's hand.

E17. Untitled commentary on Ferrier's and Soury's ideas on cortical centres
3-page unpublished typescript, undated. No marginalia.

E18. Untitled commentary on vestibular function
7-page unpublished typescript, undated. Corrections in Hughlings Jackson's hand.

E19. Out-going or in-going current?
Printed for private circulation. Labelled "Not to be returned." Dated June 6, 1904. Second copy, first copy in box 3.

E20. Untitled commentary on the cerebellum in cetacea and birds.
Unpublished typescript, labelled "For private circulation". Dated July 24, 1906. Corrections in Hughlings Jackson's hand.

Appendix 2

E21. Untitled commentary on the factors of evolution.
3-page unpublished typescript, undated. No marginalia.

E22. Tetanus-like seizures (and cerebellar rigidity?) in an infant
Typescript, much like the case published with Stephen Mackenzie. Undated. Corrections in Hughlings Jackson's hand.

E23. Untitled commentary on swearing.
1-page unpublished typescript, undated. Correction in Hughlings Jackson's hand.

E24. Untitled commentary on chest movements in hemiplegia.
2-page unpublished typescript, labelled "(From first note book, pp. 193–4)". Dated September 24, 1903. No marginalia.

E25. Untitled commentary on bulbar fits.
1-page typescript, undated, no marginalia.

E26. Untitled quotation from Maudsley's "The physiology of mind".
1-page unpublished typescript. No commentary.

E27. Loose collection of single unconnected pages of Hughlings Jackson's corrections.

Index

In the sub-headings of this index, John Hughlings Jackson's name is abbreviated to JHJ. The journals in which his publications appear are indexed only when mentioned in the editorial text.

A
amaurosis 37, 38, 40, 41, 42, 43, 49, 50, 54, 72
anaesthesia, effects of 132
Anderson, Tempest (William Charles Anderson's son) 4
Anderson, William Charles 4
antagonism, physiological 139
aphasia 22, 24–5, 50, 70, 124
   Broca's 25
   hemiplegia and 25, 53, 62, 95
   symptoms 23, 30, 72, 90
aphasic writing 72
apoplexy 39, 42, 56, 64, 69, 80
   causes 77, 79
Apothecaries Act (1815) 4
asphyxia 124, 132
ataxy, locomotor 46, 48, 49, 96, 98
   Friedreich's 122
   symptoms 96, 100
Atkinson, R 33, 84
auditory vertigo *see* Ménière's disease
automatism 69
autopsy reports 78, 87

B
Bain, Alexander 21, 30
Barnes, Robert 54, 59
Barnes, Stanley 33, 135
Bastian, H Charlton 112, 129
Beevor, Charles E 33, 117, 118
Bell, Charles 16
Bell–Magendie hypothesis 16
Bennett, A Hughes 115
blepharospasm 90
Bologna University 9
Brain 8, 22, 32, 33
the brain
   cerebellum 39, 58, 62, 65, 68, 90, 95, 119, 132, 137
   cerebral arteries 25, 49, 87
   cerebral lobes 42
   cerebral localization 15–21

the brain (cont'd)
   cerebral veins 64
   cerebrum 58, 132
   cortex 12–13, 17, 18, 25, 27, 102; basal ganglia and 19
   as equipotential 13–14
   functions 13–14, 25, 27
   lateralization of 14
   medulla oblongata 52, 66
   movement centres 67, 70
   pons varolii 39, 40
   striatum 13, 14, 25, 50
   syphilis and 54, 55, 59, 67, 69, 73, 74, 89, 95
   see also cerebral ...
brain abscesses/cysts 37, 68, 124
brain disease 42, 46, 50, 64, 80, 83, 95, 96, 97, 99, 100, 112, 115
   recovery from 101
brain lesions 86, 89
brain/mind relationship *see* concomitance doctrine
brain surgery 110
brain tumours 27, 46, 50, 62, 63, 65, 66, 67, 68, 71, 72, 73, 74, 77, 84, 87, 95, 100, 102, 118, 137
   convulsions and 102, 107
   diagnosis 70
   haemorrhage from 58
   removal of 113, 116
Bravais, François 15
breathing difficulties 124
Bright, Richard 14
Bright's disease 27
British Association for the Advancement of Science 16, 54, 55
British Medical Association (BMA) 29–30, 62, 102, 117
British Medical Journal (BMJ) 7, 11, 20, 28, 32, 33
Broadbent, Sir William 136
   JHJ's obituary by 138
   his Hughlings Jackson lecture (1903) 30, 31
Broca, Paul 7
Broca's aphasia 25

Index

Brown-Séquard, Charles Edouard 6, 9, 25
   his cases 39, 40
   JHJ and 6, 9
   working methods 9
Bucknill, John Charles 8
Buzzard, Thomas 90, 96, 97, 98, 99, 102

C
cancer 112
Cartesian philosophy 13–14
cataracts 118
cerebral apoplexy 69
cerebral haemorrhage 50, 56, 62, 78
cerebral paresis/paralysis 90, 137
   see also brain ...
cerebral pathology 65, 66, 67, 68, 71, 73, 74, 77
Chambers, Robert: *Vestiges of the natural history of creation* 29
Charcot, Jean-Martin 15, 27, 72
chemistry, JHJ's interest in 13
chloroform, effects of 132
cholera epidemic, London (1866) 7
chorea 42, 45, 46, 51, 52, 70, 76, 81
   causes 108
   in a dog 64
   embolic theory of 86
   hemi-chorea 55
   in pregnancy 54, 55, 59
Clarke, J Lockhart 31, 46, 52, 66
clinical neurophysiology 3
   evolutionary 3, 8, 19–20, 30, 106, 112, 113
Clinical Society of London 60, 62, 112
   Transactions 32
cocaine use 124
cold, sensation of 139
Collier, James S 33, 132
Colman, Walter S 33, 131
compensation principle, of the nervous system 26–7
concomitance doctrine 7, 15, 20–23, 24, 30
convulsions 12–14, 17, 53, 56, 60, 61, 64, 70, 76, 110, 119, 135
   brain tumours and 102, 107
   epileptiform *see* epileptiform ...
   partial 64, 69, 78, 79, 80, 81, 83, 97, 102
   syphilis and 89
   tongue-biting in 60
   unilateral 12, 14, 54, 55

cramp, treadler's 121
Crichton-Browne, James 8

D
Dade, Elizabeth *see* Jackson, Elizabeth Dade
Darwin, Charles: *On the origin of species* 19, 28
deafness *see* hearing loss
Descartes, René *see* Cartesian philosophy
diphtheria 27
Donders, [Frans Cornelis] 103
drunkenness 62, 73
Du Bois-Reymond, Emil 30
Dunsmure, [James] 127

E
the ear, diseases of 68, 69, 75, 87, 104, 124
   see also hearing loss
Edinburgh Medical Journal 32
Edinburgh University 9
education, JHJ on physiological aspects of 64
embolism 25, 108
Epidemiological Society 102
epilepsy 12–13, 45, 58, 68, 70, 74, 75, 77, 78, 81, 83, 84, 85, 86, 115, 118, 125, 126
   actions performed during/after 84, 87, 88
   causes 12, 13, 19, 41
   diagnosis 8, 92, 93
   effects of *see* post-epileptic states *below*
   focal 3, 8; *see also* Jacksonian *below*
   in guinea-pigs 110, 114
   hearing loss and 84, 125
   inverted compensation concept in 26–7
   Jacksonian 8, 13–15, 17, 18, 27
   mental disease and 82, 83, 116, 117
   migraine and 80
   partial 8
   post-epileptic states 22, 23, 98, 99, 116, 117
   symptoms 12, 14, 40, 41, 72, 84, 96, 117, 125, 131, 132, 133
   syphilis and 37
epileptic aphemia 43
epileptic discharge concept 12–13
epileptic mania 72, 79
epileptiform amaurosis 56, 72
epileptiform convulsions/seizures 40, 41, 43, 51, 52, 58, 63, 69, 70, 90, 97, 99, 100
   effects of 96, 97
   symptoms 44, 48

Index

epileptiform convulsions/seizures (cont'd)
  unilateral 44
ether, effects of 132
evolutionary neurophysiology 3, 8, 19–20, 30, 106, 112, 113, 114
  of the unconscious 21–4
the eye 104, 124, 139
  hemiplegia, effects of 58, 125, 132
  lateral deviation of 48, 58, 125
  locomotor ataxy and 96, 100
  optic thalamus 50
  rotation of 99, 103
  see also ophthalmology; optic neuritis; vision
eye examinations 27, 42
eyelid, innervation of 124

F

facial monoplegia 112
facial palsy 12
Faraday, Michael 12
Ferrier, David 8, 30, 78, 79, 80, 81, 83, 89
fits 127, 135
  see also epilepsy
Flourens, Pierre 13–14
focal epilepsy/lesion 3, 8, 17
  see also Jacksonian epilepsy
Friedreich's ataxy 122
fright, effects of 46

G

Gall, Franz Josef 9
Galloway, James 33, 122
gastric problems 98
Glasgow University 9
Gowers, [William R] 33, 104, 108
Graves's disease 111
Greenblatt, Samuel H 31
Gunn, Marcus 33

H

haemorrhagic infarction see pulmonary apoplexy
Hall, Marshall 16
Hamilton, William 30
Harveian Society 49, 92, 97, 110,
  JHJ as president 8
head injuries, epilepsy caused by 41
hearing loss 30, 48, 65, 75, 80
  see also the ear

heart disease 11, 69
  valvular 24–5, 43, 45
heat, sensation of 139
hemianaesthesia 78
hemianopsia 112
hemikinesis 79
hemiplegia 7, 11, 12, 17, 25, 43, 45, 46, 69, 73, 74, 78, 84, 87, 125
  aphasia and 25, 53, 62, 95
  double 122
  eyes, effects on 58, 125, 132
  recovery from 73, 76, 121
  speech loss and 43, 46, 49, 73
  symptoms 122, 132
  syphilis and 63
  temporary 40, 90, 97
Hitzig, Eduard 8, 13, 78, 79, 80, 81, 83
Holmes, Gordon 31
Horsley, Victor 110
Hughlings, John (JHJ's maternal grandfather) 3
Hughlings, Sarah see Jackson, Sarah
Hughlings Jackson, John see Jackson, John Hughlings
Hunterian Society 64, 121, 122
Hutchinson, Jonathan 5, 6
  JHJ and 5–6, 7, 28, 34
  on JHJ's crisis of intention 28
  as a medical reporter 6, 33
Huxley, Thomas Henry 21, 30

I

ideas, as imperative 128
Illustrated London News 32
inhibition(s) 20, 115
insanity see mental disease
International Medical Congress, 1881,
  Transactions 32

J

Jackson, Elizabeth Dade (Mrs John Hughlings Jackson) (JHJ's wife) 7, 8
Jackson, James (JHJ's great-uncle) 4
Jackson, John Hughlings (JHJ)
  as an agnostic 17
  bust of, at London Hospital 138
  career 5, 6–7; his crisis of intention 28
  character 24, 28, 34
  his collaborators 31–2

Index

Jackson, John Hughlings (JHJ) (cont'd)
  death 9; obituary by Sir William Broadbent 138
  education 3, 4, 28; medical 4, 6; surgical 4–5
  experimental work 27, 42
  family 3–4, 5, 7, 28, 29
  financial position 5, 28
  honorary degrees 9
  impact/influence 3, 7, 8
  lectures 7, 10, 27, 29–30, 69, 80, 92, 95, 96, 122, 131, 136; Bowman 27, 108, 109; Croonian 8, 9, 20, 22, 106, 107; Goulstonian 7, 9, 12, 57; at London Hospital 6, 10; Lumleian 8–9, 13, 119
  life 3–9, 28
  in London 5–6, 28
  marriage 7
  as a medical reporter 6, 9, 33
  philosophy, his interest in 28–30
  as a physician 3, 6, 29, 34
  reading habits 29
  reputation *see* impact/influence *above*
  reviews by 61, 108
  testimonials to 126, 127
  his writings 29, 30–34; reviews of 74, 75, 83
  in York/Yorkshire 3, 4, 5, 13, 16
Jackson, Samuel (JHJ's father) 3, 5
  financial position 5, 28
Jackson, Sarah (née Hughlings) (JHJ's mother) 3, 4
Jackson, Thomas (JHJ's brother) 4, 5, 28
Jacksonian compensation *see* compensation principle
Jacksonian epilepsy 8, 13–15, 17, 18, 27
joking, psychology of 113, 116
Journal of Mental Science 32
Journal of Psychological Medicine and Mental Pathology 32

K
keratitis, interstitial 42
knee-jerks 121, 122, 124, 125, 126, 129
Kussmaul, [Adolf] 126

L
Lancet 7, 20, 32, 33
language 30, 48
  intellectual/emotional 25, 48
  physiology of 54, 55

language (cont'd)
  spoken *see* speech ...
  written 25, 49, 125
language centre, in the brain 7, 25
Laycock, Thomas 4, 21, 30
  JHJ and 4, 16
  on reflex actions 16, 17
Leeds University 9
Leibniz, Gottfried Wilhelm 21, 30
Lewes, G H 22
London Hospital 54, 58, 60, 62, 63, 64, 65, 66, 67, 68, 69, 72, 73, 74, 75, 77, 78, 79, 80, 81, 83, 84, 86, 87, 89, 90, 91
  JHJ at 5, 7, 52, 53; as pathology lecturer 6
  JHJ's lecture at 10
  JHJ's retirement from 9; testimonial to 127
  presents JHJ with gold watch 7
London Hospital Gazette 32
London Hospital *Reports* 7, 10, 24, 32
London Medical Record 10

M
Mackenzie, Frederick 52
Mackenzie, Morell 33, 60
Magendie, François 16
materialism 29, 30
Maudsley, Henry 49
Maunder, Mr (of London Hospital) 68
medical education/training 4–5
Medical Examiner 32
Medical Mirror 32
Medical Press and Circular 19, 32, 33
Medical Record 33
Medical Society of London 102, 108, 110, 112, 113, 116, 117, 121
  JHJ's Annual Oration to (1877) 27
  JHJ as president 8, 34
  Proceedings 32
  Transactions 33
medical specialization, bias against 9
Medical Times and Gazette 6, 14, 20, 25, 32, 33
Mendel's hypothesis 123
Ménière's disease 65, 72, 80, 93, 96, 136
meningitis, tubercular 78
mental disease 19, 21, 30, 48, 125
  causes 49
  epilepsy and 82, 83, 116, 117
  see also the mind

Index

Mercier, Charles 24, 115
metaphysics
  Pierre Flourens on 14
  JHJ's rejection of 29
  of the nervous system 16, 17, 18, 21, 24, 29–30
Metropolitan Free Hospital, London 6
migraine 80, 102
Mill, John Stuart 21, 30
the mind 23, 123
  concomitance doctrine of 7, 15, 20–23, 24, 30
  post-epileptic behaviour and 22, 23
  structure of 21–2
  the unconscious 21–4
  see also mental disease
Money, Dr Angel 108
monoplegia 112
  see also paralysis
Moorfields Eye Hospital, *see* Royal London Ophthalmic Hospital
Müller, Frederick Max 30
muscular atrophy 52
muscular sense concept 112

N

National Hospital for the Paralysed and Epileptic, London 6, 9, 34, 43, 49, 55, 58, 59, 60, 63, 65, 71, 72, 74, 78, 80, 84, 96, 133
  JHJ at 6; his retirement from 9
  JHJ's bust in hall of 138
necrosis, focal 3
nervous dissolution concept 8, 19, 20, 22–3, 79, 97, 98, 99, 102, 103, 104, 105, 106, 112, 113, 114
nervous system 54, 55, 56, 57, 58, 83, 94, 127
  compensation principle of 26–7
  concomitance doctrine of 7, 15, 20–23, 24, 30
  evolutionary theory of 3, 8, 19–24, 30, 106, 112, 113, 114
  functions/functioning of 3, 7, 8, 9–10, 11, 16
  JHJ's neurological method 9–11
  metaphysics of 16, 17, 18, 21, 24, 29, 30
  as a sensorimotor machine 15, 16–17, 18, 20
  structure 3, 8, 9–10, 15, 18, 19–20, 26
  theories of 9–10
  tonic inhibition concept 20
  the unconscious 21–2
  see also spinal cord ...

nervous system, diseases of 44, 51, 52, 57, 58, 60, 63, 68, 77, 79, 84, 86, 102, 117, 127, 136
  causes 25, 49
  cerebral localization in 15–21
  diagnosis 3, 7, 8, 9–10, 13–14; somatopic representation on 13, 14, 15, 17–18
  ear disease and 87
  ophthalmology and 27, 108, 110
  recovery from 25–7, 39, 41, 73, 76
  symptoms 3, 9–10, 11, 25, 48, 50, 129; negative/positive 3, 19, 20, 23
  see also individual conditions
neuritis, optic 53, 54, 55, 60, 62, 63, 68, 76, 91, 97, 98, 99, 100; double optic 85
neurological fragments (JHJ's) 122, 123, 124, 125, 126, 127, 129, 130, 132, 135, 139
Neurological Society of London 112
  JHJ as president 9
  Hughlings Jackson Lecture 9, 131
neurophysiology *see* clinical neurophysiology

O

Obstetrical Society of London 54
Transactions 33
odour, as symptom of epileptiform seizures 44, 53, 117
  see also smell, sense of
Ophthalmic Review 33
Ophthalmological Society of the United Kingdom 33, 96, 97, 98, 99, 104, 111, 118
  Bowman Lecture 27, 108, 109
  JHJ as president 8, 27, 117, 118, 120
  Transactions 32
ophthalmology 27, 37, 59, 72, 81, 88, 89, 108, 110, 117, 118
  examinations during sleep 42
  see also eye ... ; vision
ophthalmoplegia 123
ophthalmoscopes 39, 42, 50, 51, 53, 54, 62, 93, 96
opium poisoning 124
optic neuritis 53, 54, 55, 60, 62, 63, 68, 91, 97, 98, 99, 100
  double 85
  recovery from 76
Owen, Richard 10

Index

P
Paget, Sir James 4, 9, 127
palsies 51, 52, 60, 67
paralysis 5, 38, 45, 112, 115, 116, 117, 118, 121, 139
  causes 12, 16, 97
  cerebral 90, 137
  hemiplegia *see* hemiplegia
  partial 17–18, 40
  in Pott's disease 110
  recovery from 25–7
  spinal cord injuries and 129, 130
  syphilis and 37, 40, 112
  Todd's 29
  of the tongue 66, 90, 110, 112
pathology 102
  cerebral 65, 66, 67, 71, 72, 73, 74, 77
Paton, Leslie 139
Patton, J 33
philosophy
  metaphysics 14, 16, 17, 18, 21, 24, 29–30
  in Victorian England 29
phonographic recordings, of abnormal speech 121
phrenology 9, 10
physiological antagonism 139
pneumonia 126
poliomyelitis 98
The Polyclinic 32
Popular Science Monthly 33
potassium, iodine of 42
Pott's disease, paraplegia in 110
pregnancy, chorea in 54, 55, 59
psychology 114
  of joking 113, 116
ptosis, congenital 124
pulmonary apoplexy 69
pyaemia 54

R
reading, loss of ability to 49
recordings *see* phonographic recordings
reflex actions 16, 17, 108
La Revue Scientifique de la France ... 33
Reynolds, J R: *A system of medicine* 32, 56
rheumatic heart disease 11
rigidity 119, 132
Rivers, W H R 33, 121
Robertson, [Alexander] 86

Rockefeller Medical Library, Institute of Neurology, University College London
  JHJ's pamphlets held by 140–45
  JHJ's unpublished writings held by 146–50
Ross, James 108
Royal College of Physicians 6
  Croonian lecture 8, 9, 20, 22, 30, 106, 107
  Goulstonian lecture 7, 9, 12, 57
  JHJ as Censor 9; as Council member 9; as Fellow 7
  Lumleian lecture 8–9, 13, 119
Royal College of Surgeons 4, 5, 6
Royal London Ophthalmic Hospital, JHJ at 5, 6, 7, 27
  Reports 7, 32
Royal Medical and Chirurgical Society 81, 108
  Medico-Chirurgical Transactions 33
Royal Society, JHJ as Fellow 8
Russell, James S Risien 24, 33, 124, 125

S
St Andrews Medical Graduates' Association
  Transactions 7–8, 12, 32
St Andrews University MD degree 6, 7
St Bartholomew's Hospital 4–5
Savage, Dr [G H] 115
scarlet fever 39
scientific neurology *see* nervous system ...
sensorimotor machine, nervous system as 15, 16–17, 18, 20
sex, diseases of the nervous system and 49
Sherrington, [Charles Scott] 129
sight *see* eye ...; ophthalmology; vision
Singer, H Douglas 33, 135
smell, sense of 48, 74, 118, 132, 133
smoking *see* tobacco smoking
somatopic representation, in diagnostic neurology 13, 14, 15, 17–18
the soul *see* metaphysics
spasm 51, 52, 96, 135
speech *see* language
speech defects 64, 90, 93, 94, 95
  phonographic recordings of 121
speech loss 25, 30, 48, 49, 67, 72, 125, 126
  hemiplegia and 43, 45, 46, 49, 73
  tongue, paralysis of 66, 110
  vocal cord palsy and 67, 110
Spencer, Herbert 19, 21, 29, 30

156

Index

spinal cord 10, 16
spinal cord disease 39, 40, 52, 99, 124
spinal cord injuries 39, 40, 129, 130
   symptoms 104
Sprengel's shoulder 134
Stewart, Purves 33, 132, 133
Suggestions for studying diseases of the nervous system . . . (privately printed pamphlet by JHJ) 10
Sunderland, H 83
super-venosity 122
surgical training 4–5
syphilis 38, 63, 67, 69, 89
   the brain, effects on 54, 55, 69, 74, 89
   congenital 77
   epilepsy and 37
   inherited 56, 58
   intercranial 59, 67, 73, 95
   paralysis and 37, 40, 112
   symptoms 27, 77, 80, 112
syringomyelus 122

T

taste, sense of 74
Taylor, James 93, 121, 122, 125
   JHJ and 8, 30, 33
   Selected writings of John Hughlings Jackson (ed.) 31–2
testes 48
tetanus 90, 91
Thompson, Tatham 118
thrombosis of syphilitic arteries 69
tobacco smoking 49
Todd, Robert Bentley 5, 9, 12, 86
   JHJ and 9, 12, 17
   working methods 9
Todd's paralysis 29
tongue, paralysis of 66, 90, 112
   see also speech . . .; taste
tonic inhibition concept 20
treadler's cramp 121

tubercular meningitis 78
Tuke, Hack 128
Tyndall, John 30

U

the unconscious 22–3, 24
   definition 23
   evolutionary theory of 21–4

V

vertigo 27, 104
   auditory (Ménière's disease) 65, 72, 80, 93, 96, 136
   causes 69
vision 42, 43, 47, 48, 67
   coloured 37, 41, 72
   see also eye . . .; ophthalmology
vocal chord palsy *see* speech loss

W

Walshe, Francis 31
Wernicke, [Carl] 126
West Riding Lunatic Asylum Medical Reports 32
Woodman, W Bathurst 74
word-blindness 125, 126
Worshipful Society of Apothecaries 4, 5, 6
writing 25
   inability to write 49, 125

Y

York County Hospital 4
York Dispensary 5
York Medical School 4, 13, 16
York Medical Society 5
   Minute Book 12

Z

Zoological Society 16